How the Immune
System Works

I dedicate this book to my sweetheart, my best friend, and my wife: Vicki Sompayrac.

How the Immune System Works

FIFTH EDITION

Lauren Sompayrac, PhD

WILEY Blackwell

Registered office: John Wiley & Sons, Ltd, The Atrium, Southern Gate, Chichester, West Sussex, PO19 8SQ, UK

Editorial offices: 9600 Garsington Road, Oxford, OX4 2DQ, UK
    1606 Golden Aspen Drive, Suites 103 and 104, Ames, Iowa 50010, USA

For details of our global editorial offices, for customer services and for information about how to apply for permission to reuse the copyright material in this book please see our website at www.wiley.com/wiley-blackwell

Library of Congress Cataloging-in-Publication Data
Sompayrac, Lauren, author.
  How the immune system works / Lauren Sompayrac. -- Fifth edition.
    p. ; cm.
  Includes index.
  ISBN 978-1-118-99777-2 (pbk.)
  I. Title.
  [DNLM: 1. Immune System--physiology. 2. Immune System--anatomy & histology. 3. Immune System--physiopathology. 4. Immunity--physiology. QW 504]
  QR181
  616.07′9--dc23
                                     2015015315
A catalogue record for this book is available from the British Library.

Wiley also publishes its books in a variety of electronic formats. Some content that appears in print may not be available in electronic books.

Cover image and figure on page 2 used with permission from Lennart Nilsson/TT.

Set in 9.5/13 in Palatino LT Std by Aptara, India
Printed in Singapore

1 2016

Contents

This book is neither a comprehensive text nor an exam-review tool. It is an overview of the immune system, designed to give anyone who is learning immunology a feel for how the system fits together.

The immune system is a "team effort," involving many different players who work together to provide a powerful defense against invaders. Focusing in on one player at a time makes it hard to understand the game. Here we view the action from the grandstands to get a wide-angle picture of what the immune system is all about.

The innate immune system is a "hard-wired" defense that has evolved over millions of years to recognize pathogens that commonly infect humans. It provides a rapid and powerful response against "everyday" invaders.

B cells and the antibodies they produce are part of the adaptive immune system. This defense evolves during our own lifetime to protect us against invaders that we, personally, have never encountered before.

T cells, another weapon of the adaptive immune system, only recognize invaders which are "properly presented" by specialized antigen presenting cells. This feature keeps these important cells focused on the particular attackers which they are able to defend against.

Before they can spring into action, T cells must be activated. This requirement helps insure that only useful weapons will be mobilized.

Once they have been activated, helper T cells orchestrate the immune response, and killer T cells destroy infected cells.

Acknowledgments

I would like to thank the following people, whose critical comments on earlier editions were most helpful: Drs. Mark Dubin, Linda Clayton, Dan Tenen, Jim Cook, Tom Mitchell, Lanny Rosenwasser, and Eric Martz. Thanks also go to Diane Lorenz, who illustrated the first and second editions, and whose wonderful artwork still can be found in this book. Finally, I wish to thank Vicki Sompayrac, whose wise suggestions helped make this book more readable, and whose editing was invaluable in preparing the final manuscript.

How to Use This Book

I wrote *How the Immune System Works* because I couldn't find a book that would give my students an overall view of the immune system. Sure, there are as many good, thick textbooks as a person might have money to buy, but these are crammed with every possible detail. There are also lots of "review books" that are great if you want a summary of what you've already learned – but they won't teach you immunology. What was missing was a short book that tells, in simple language, how the immune system fits together – a book that presents the big picture of the immune system, without the jargon and the details.

How the Immune System Works is written in the form of "lectures," because I want to talk to you directly, just as if we were together in a classroom. Although Lecture 1 is a light-hearted overview, meant to give you a running start at the subject, you'll soon discover that this is not "baby immunology." *How the Immune System Works* is a concept-driven analysis of how the immune system players work together to protect us from disease – and, most importantly, why they do it this way.

In Lectures 2 through 10, I focus more closely on the individual players and their roles. These lectures are short, so you probably can read them all in a couple of afternoons. In fact, **I strongly suggest that you begin by reading quickly through Lectures 1–10.** The whole idea is to get an overall view of the subject, and if you read one lecture a week, that won't happen. Don't "study" these 10 lectures your first time through. Don't even bother with the Thought Questions at the end of each lecture. Just rip through them. Then, once you have a "feel" for

the system, go back and spend a bit more time with these same 10 lectures to get a clearer understanding of the "hows and whys."

In Lectures 11–15, I discuss the intestinal immune system, vaccines, allergies, autoimmune disease, the AIDS virus, and cancer. These lectures will let you "practice" what you have learned in the earlier lectures by examining real-world examples of the immune system at work. So after you have gone through Lectures 1–10 twice, I'd suggest you read these last five lectures. When you do, I think you'll be amazed by how much you now understand about the immune system.

As you read, you will encounter passages highlighted in blue, and words that are highlighted in red. These highlights are to alert you to important concepts and terms. They also will help you review a lecture quickly, once you have read it through.

In some settings, *How the Immune System Works* will serve as the main text for the immunology section of a larger course. For a semester-long undergraduate or graduate immunology course, your professor may use this book as a companion to a comprehensive textbook. As your course proceeds, reviewing the appropriate lectures in *How the Immune System Works* will help you keep the big picture in focus as the details are filled in. It's really easy to get lost in the details.

No matter how your professor may choose to use this book, you should keep one important point in mind: I didn't write *How the Immune System Works* for your professor. This book is for you!

An Overview

INTRODUCTION

Immunology is a difficult subject for several reasons. First, there are lots of details, and sometimes these details get in the way of understanding the concepts. To get around this problem, we're going to concentrate on the big picture. It will be easy for you to find the details somewhere else. Another difficulty in learning immunology is that there is an exception to every rule. Immunologists love these exceptions, because they give clues as to how the immune system functions. But for now, we're just going to learn the rules. Oh, sure, we'll come upon exceptions from time to time, but we won't dwell on them. Our goal is to examine the immune system, stripped to its essence.

A third difficulty in studying immunology is that our knowledge of the immune system is still evolving. As you'll see, there are many unanswered questions, and some of the things that seem true today will be proven false tomorrow. I'll try to give you a feeling for the way things stand now, and from time to time I'll discuss what immunologists speculate may be true. But keep in mind that although I'll try to be straight with you, some of the things I'll tell you will change in the future – maybe even by the time you read this!

Although these three features make studying immunology difficult, I think the main reason immunology is such a tough subject is that the immune system is a "team effort" that involves many different players interacting with each other. Imagine you're watching a football game on TV, and the camera is isolated on one player, say, the tight end. You see him run at full speed down the field, and then stop. It doesn't seem to make any sense. Later, however, you see the same play on the big screen, and now you understand. That tight end took two defenders with him down the field, leaving the running back uncovered to catch the pass and run for a touchdown. The immune system is a lot like a football team. It's a network of players who cooperate to get things done, and focusing on a single player doesn't make much sense. You need an overall view. That's the purpose of this first lecture, which you might call "turbo immunology." Here, I'm going to take you on a quick tour of the immune system, so you can get a feeling for how it all fits together. Then in the next lectures, we'll go back and take a closer look at the individual players and their interactions.

PHYSICAL BARRIERS

Our first line of defense against invaders consists of physical barriers, and to cause real trouble, viruses, bacteria, parasites, and fungi must penetrate these shields. Although we tend to think of our skin as the main barrier, the area covered by our skin is only about 2 square meters. In contrast, the area covered by the mucous membranes that line our digestive, respiratory, and reproductive tracts measures about 400 square meters – an area about as big as two tennis courts. The main point here is that there is a large perimeter which must be defended.

THE INNATE IMMUNE SYSTEM

Any invader that breaches the physical barrier of skin or mucosa is greeted by the **innate immune system** – our second line of defense. Immunologists call this system "innate" because it is a defense that all animals just naturally seem to have. Indeed, some of the weapons of the innate immune system have been around for more than 500 million years. Let me give you an example of how this amazing innate system works.

Imagine you are getting out of your hot tub, and as you step onto the deck, you get a large splinter in your big toe. On that splinter are many bacteria, and within a few hours you'll notice (unless you had a lot to drink in that hot tub!) that the area around where the splinter entered is red and swollen. These are indications that your innate immune system has kicked in. In your tissues are roving bands of white blood cells that defend you against attack. To us, tissue looks pretty solid, but that's because we're so big. To a cell, tissue looks somewhat like a sponge with holes through which individual cells can move rather freely. One of the defender cells that is stationed in your tissues is the most famous innate immune system player of them all: the **macrophage**. If you are a bacterium, a macrophage is the last cell you want to see after your ride on that splinter! Here is an electron micrograph showing a macrophage about to devour a bacterium.

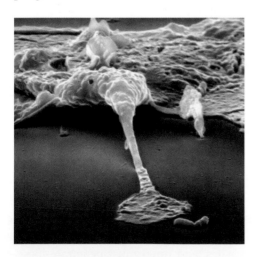

You will notice that this macrophage isn't just waiting until it bumps into the bacterium, purely by chance. No, this macrophage actually has sensed the presence of the bacterium, and is reaching out a "foot" to grab it. But how does a macrophage know that a bacterium is out there? The answer is that macrophages have antennae (receptors) on their surface which are tuned to recognize "danger molecules" characteristic of common microbial invaders. For example, the membranes that surround bacteria are made up of certain fats and carbohydrates that normally are not found in the human body. Some of these foreign molecules represent "find me and eat me" signals for macrophages. And when macrophages detect danger molecules, they begin to crawl toward the microbe which is emitting these molecules.

When it encounters a bacterium, a macrophage first engulfs it in a pouch (vesicle) called a **phagosome**. The vesicle containing the bacterium is then taken inside the macrophage, where it fuses with another vesicle termed a **lysosome**. Lysosomes contain powerful chemicals and enzymes which can destroy bacteria. In fact, these agents are so destructive that they would kill the macrophage itself if they were released inside it. That's why they are kept in vesicles. Using this clever strategy, the macrophage can destroy an invader without "shooting itself in the foot." This whole process is called **phagocytosis**, and this series of snapshots shows how it happens.

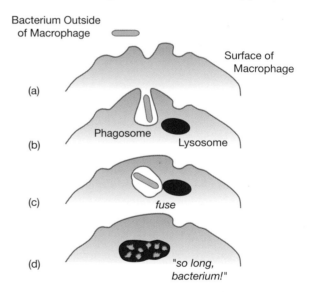

Macrophages have been around for a very long time. In fact, the ingestion technique macrophages employ is simply a refinement of the strategy that amoebas use to feed themselves – and amoebas have roamed Earth for about 2.5 billion years. So why is this creature called a macrophage? "Macro," of course, means large – and a macrophage is a large cell. "Phage" comes from a Greek word meaning "to eat." So a macrophage is a big eater. In fact, in addition to defending against invaders, the macrophage functions as a garbage collector. It will eat almost anything. Immunologists can take advantage of this appetite by feeding macrophages iron filings. Then, using a small magnet, they can separate macrophages from other cells in a cell mixture. Really!

Where do macrophages come from? Macrophages and all the other blood cells in your body are made in the bone marrow, where they descend from self-renewing cells called **stem cells** – the cells from which all the blood cells "stem." By self-renewing, I mean that when a stem cell grows and divides into two daughter cells, it does a "one for me, one for you" thing in which some of the daughter cells go back to being stem cells, and some of the daughters go on to become mature blood cells. This strategy of continuous self-renewal insures that there will always be blood stem cells in reserve to carry on the process of making mature blood cells.

As each daughter cell matures, it has to make choices that determine which type of blood cell it will become when it grows up. As you can imagine, these choices are not random, but are carefully controlled to make sure you have enough of each kind of blood cell. For example, some daughter cells become red blood cells, which capture oxygen in the lungs and transport it to all parts of the body. In fact, our stem cell "factories" must turn out more than two million new red blood cells each second to replace those lost due to normal wear and tear. Other descendants of a stem cell may become macrophages, neutrophils, or other types of "white" blood cells. And just as white wine really isn't white, these cells aren't white either. They are colorless, but biologists use the term "white" to indicate that they lack hemoglobin, and therefore are not red. Here is a figure showing some of the many different kinds of blood cells a stem cell can become.

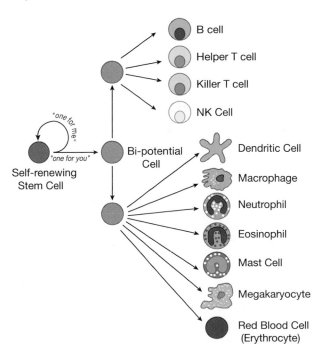

When the cells which will mature into macrophages first exit the bone marrow and enter the blood stream, they are called **monocytes**. All in all, you have about two billion of these cells circulating in your blood at any one time. This may seem a little creepy, but you can be very glad they are there. Without them, you'd be in deep trouble. Monocytes remain in the blood for an average of about three days. During this time they travel to the capillaries – which represent the "end of the line" for blood vessels – looking for a crack between the endothelial cells that line the inside of the capillaries. These endothelial cells are shaped like shingles, and by sticking a foot between them, a monocyte can leave the blood, enter the tissues, and mature into a macrophage. Once in the tissues, most macrophages just hang out, do their garbage collecting thing, and wait for you to get that splinter so they can do some real work.

When macrophages eat the bacteria on that splinter in your foot, they give off chemicals which increase the flow of blood to the vicinity of the wound. The buildup of blood in this area is what makes your toe red. Some of these chemicals also cause the cells that line the blood vessels to contract, leaving spaces between them so that fluid from the capillaries can leak out into the tissues. It is this fluid which causes the swelling. In addition, chemicals released by macrophages can stimulate nerves in the tissues that surround the splinter, sending pain signals to your brain to alert you that something isn't quite right in the area of your big toe.

During their battle with bacteria, macrophages produce and give off (secrete) proteins called **cytokines**. These are hormone-like messengers which facilitate communication between cells of the immune system. Some of these cytokines alert monocytes and other immune system cells traveling in nearby capillaries that the battle is on, and encourage these cells to exit the blood to help fight the rapidly multiplying bacteria. Pretty soon, you have a vigorous "inflammatory" response going on in your toe, as the innate immune system battles to eliminate the invaders.

So here's the strategy: You have a large perimeter to defend, so you station sentinels (macrophages) to check for invaders. When these sentinels encounter the enemy, they send out signals (cytokines) that recruit more defenders to the site of the battle. The macrophages then do their best to hold off the invaders until reinforcements arrive. Because the innate response involves warriors like macrophages, which are programmed to recognize many common invaders, your innate immune system usually responds so quickly that the battle is over in just a few days.

There are other players on the innate team. For example, in addition to the **professional phagocytes** like macrophages, which make it their business to eat invaders, the innate system also includes the complement proteins that can punch holes in bacteria, and natural killer (NK) cells that are able to destroy bacteria, parasites, virus-infected cells, and some cancer cells. We will talk more about the macrophage's innate system teammates in the next lecture.

THE ADAPTIVE IMMUNE SYSTEM

About 99% of all animals get along just fine with only natural barriers and the innate immune system to protect them. However, for vertebrates like us, Mother Nature laid on a third level of defense: the **adaptive immune system**. This is a defense system which actually can adapt to protect us against almost any invader. One of the first clues that the adaptive immune system existed came back in the 1790s when Edward Jenner began vaccinating the English against smallpox virus. In those days, smallpox was a major health problem. Hundreds of thousands of people died from this disease, and many more were horribly disfigured. What Jenner observed was that milkmaids frequently contracted a disease called cowpox which caused lesions on their hands that looked similar to the sores caused by the smallpox virus. Jenner also noted that milkmaids who had contracted cowpox almost never got smallpox (which, it turns out, is caused by a close relative of the cowpox virus).

So Jenner decided to conduct a daring experiment. He collected pus from the sores of a milkmaid who had cowpox, and used it to inoculate a little boy named James Phipps. Later, when Phipps was re-inoculated with pus from the sores of a person infected with smallpox, he did not contract that disease. In Latin, the word for cow is *vacca* – which explains where we get the word vaccine. History makes out the hero in this affair to be Edward Jenner, but I think the real hero that day was the young boy. Imagine having this big man approach you with a large needle and a tube full of pus! Although this isn't the sort of thing that could be done today, we can be thankful that Jenner's experiment was a success, because it paved the way for vaccinations that have saved countless lives.

Smallpox virus was not something humans encountered regularly. So Jenner's experiment showed that if the human immune system were given time to prepare, it could produce weapons that could provide protection against an intruder it had never seen before. Importantly, the smallpox vaccination only protected against smallpox or closely related viruses such as cowpox. James Phipps was still able to get mumps, measles, and the rest. This is one of the hallmarks of the adaptive immune system: It adapts to defend against specific invaders.

Antibodies and B cells

Eventually, immunologists determined that immunity to smallpox was conferred by special proteins that circulated in the blood of immunized individuals. These proteins were named **antibodies**, and the agent that caused the antibodies to be made was called an **antigen** – in this case, the cowpox virus. Here's a sketch that shows the prototype antibody, **immunoglobulin G (IgG)**.

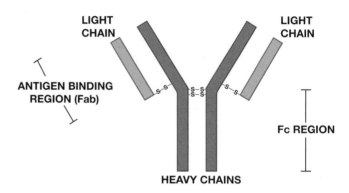

As you can see, an IgG antibody molecule is made up of two pairs of two different proteins, the **heavy chain (Hc)** and the **light chain (Lc)**. Because of this structure, each molecule has two identical "hands" (**Fab regions**) that can bind to antigens. Proteins are the ideal molecules to use for constructing antibodies that can grasp attackers, because different proteins can fold up into a myriad of complex shapes.

IgG makes up about 75% of the antibodies in the blood, but there are four other classes of antibodies: **IgA**, **IgD**, **IgE**, and **IgM**. Each kind of antibody is produced by B cells – white blood cells that are born in the bone marrow, and which can mature to become antibody factories called **plasma B cells**.

In addition to having hands that can bind to an antigen, an antibody molecule also has a **constant region (Fc)** "tail" which can bind to receptors (**Fc receptors**) on the surface of cells such as macrophages. In fact, it is the special structure of the antibody Fc region that determines its **class** (e.g., IgG vs. IgA), which immune system cells it will bind to, and how it will function.

The hands of each antibody bind to a specific antigen (e.g., a protein on the surface of the smallpox virus), so in order to have antibodies available that can bind to many different antigens, many different antibody molecules are required. Now, if we want antibodies to protect us from every possible invader (and we do!), how many different antibodies would we need? Well, immunologists have made rough estimates that about 100 million should do the trick. Since each antigen-binding region of an antibody is composed of a heavy chain and a light chain, we could mix and match about 10 000 different heavy chains with 10 000 different light chains to get the 100 million different antibodies we need. However, human cells only have about 25 000 genes in all, so if each heavy or light chain protein were encoded by a different gene, most of the B cell's genetic information would be used up just to make antibodies. You see the problem.

Generating antibody diversity by modular design

The riddle of how B cells could produce the 100 million different antibodies required to protect us was solved in 1977 by Susumu Tonegawa, who received the Nobel Prize for his discovery. When Tonegawa started working on this problem, the dogma was that the DNA in every cell in the body was the same. This made perfect sense, because after an egg is fertilized, the DNA in the egg is copied. These copies are then passed down to the daughter cells, where they are copied again, and passed down to their daughters – and so on. Therefore, barring errors in copying, each of our cells should end up with the same DNA as the original, fertilized egg. Tonegawa, however, hypothesized that although this is probably true in general, there might be exceptions. His idea was that all of our B cells might start out with the same DNA, but that as these cells mature, the DNA that makes up the antibody genes might change – and these changes might be enough to generate the 100 million different antibodies we need.

Tonegawa decided to test this hypothesis by comparing the DNA sequence of the light chain from a mature B cell with the DNA sequence of the light chain from an immature B cell. Sure enough, he found that they were different, and that they were different in a very interesting way. What Tonegawa and others discovered was that the mature antibody genes are made by modular design.

In every B cell, on the chromosomes that encode the antibody heavy chain, there are multiple copies of four types of DNA modules (**gene segments**) called V, D,

J, and C. Each copy of a given module is slightly different from the other copies of that module. For example, in humans there are about 40 different V segments, about 25 different D segments, 6 different J segments, and so on. To assemble a mature heavy chain gene, each B cell chooses (more or less at random) one of each kind of gene segment, and pastes them together like this.

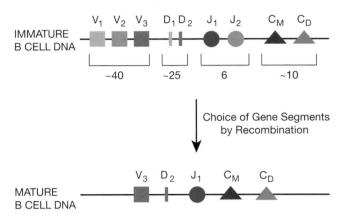

You have seen this kind of mix-and-match strategy used before to create diversity. For example, 20 different amino acids are mixed and matched to create the huge number of different proteins that our cells produce. And to create genetic diversity, the chromosomes you inherited from your mother and father are mixed and matched to make the set of chromosomes that goes into your egg or sperm cells. Once Mother Nature gets a good idea, she uses it over and over – and modular design is one of her very best ideas.

The DNA that encodes the light chain of the antibody molecule is also assembled by picking gene segments and pasting them together. Because there are so many different gene segments that can be mixed and matched, this scheme can be used to create about 10 million different antibodies – not quite enough. So, to make things even more diverse, when the gene segments are joined together, additional DNA bases are added or deleted. When this **junctional diversity** is included, there is no problem creating 100 million B cells, each with the ability to make a different antibody. The magic of this scheme is that by using modular design and junctional diversity, only a small amount of genetic information is required to create incredible antibody diversity.

Clonal selection

In the human blood stream, there is a total of about three billion B cells. This seems like a lot, but if there are 100 million different kinds of B cells (to produce the

100 million different kinds of antibodies we need for protection), this means that, on average, there will only be about 30 B cells in the blood that can produce an antibody which will bind to a given antigen (e.g., a protein on the surface of a virus). Said another way, although we have B cells in our arsenal that can deal with essentially any invader, we don't have a lot of any one kind of B cell. As a result, when we are attacked, more of the appropriate B cells must be made. Indeed, B cells are made "on demand." But how does the immune system know which B cells to make more of? The solution to this problem is one of the most elegant in all of immunology: the principle of clonal selection.

After B cells do their mix-and-match thing and paste together the modules required to form the "recipes" for their heavy and light chain antibody proteins, a relatively small number of these proteins is made – a "test batch" of antibody molecules, if you will. These tester antibodies, called **B cell receptors (BCRs)**, are transported to the surface of the B cell and are tethered there with their antigen-binding regions facing out. Each B cell has roughly 100 000 BCRs anchored on its surface, and all the BCRs on a given B cell recognize the same antigen.

The B cell receptors on the surface of a B cell act like "bait," and what they are "fishing for" is the molecule which their Fab regions have the right shape to grasp – their **cognate antigen**. Sadly, the vast majority of B cells fish in vain. For example, most of us will never be infected with the SARS virus or the AIDS virus. Consequently, those B cells in our body which could make antibodies that recognize these viruses never will find their match. It must be very frustrating for most B cells. They fish all their lives, and never catch anything!

On occasion, however, a B cell does make a catch. And when a B cell's receptors bind to its cognate antigen, that B cell is triggered to double in size and divide into two daughter cells – a process immunologists call **proliferation**. Both daughter cells then double in size and divide to produce a total of four cells, and so forth. Each cycle of cell growth and division takes about 12 hours to complete, and this period of proliferation usually lasts about a week. At the end of this time, a "clone" of roughly 20 000 identical B cells will have been produced, all of which have receptors on their surface that can recognize the same antigen. Now there are enough B cells to mount a real defense!

After the selected B cells proliferate to form this large clone, most of them begin to make antibodies in earnest. The antibodies produced by these selected B cells are slightly different from the antibody molecules displayed on their surface in that there is no "anchor" to attach them to the B cell's surface. As a result, these antibodies are transported out of the B cell and into the blood stream. One B cell, working at full capacity, can pump out about 2000 antibody molecules per second! After making this heroic effort, most of these B cells die, having worked for only about a week as antibody factories.

When you think about it, this is a marvelous strategy. First, because they employ modular design, B cells use relatively few genes to create enough different antibody molecules to recognize any possible invader. Second, B cells are made on demand. So instead of filling up our bodies with a huge number of B cells which may never be used, we begin with a relatively small number of B cells, and then select the particular B cells that will be useful against the "invader *du jour*." Once selected, the B cells proliferate rapidly to produce a large clone of B cells whose antibodies are guaranteed to be useful against the invader. Third, after the clone of B cells has grown sufficiently large, most of these cells become antibody factories which manufacture huge quantities of the very antibodies that are right to defend against the invader. Finally, when the intruder has been conquered, most of the B cells die. As a result, we don't fill up with B cells that are appropriate to defend against yesterday's invader, but which would be useless against the enemy that attacks us tomorrow. I love this system!

What antibodies do

Interestingly, although antibodies are very important in the defense against invaders, they really don't kill anything. Their job is to plant the "kiss of death" on an invader – to tag it for destruction. If you go to a fancy wedding, you'll usually pass through a receiving line before you are allowed to enjoy the champagne and cake. Of course, one of the functions of this receiving line is to introduce everyone to the bride and groom. But the other function is to be sure no outsiders are admitted to the celebration. As you pass through the line, you will be screened by someone who is familiar with all the invited guests. If she finds that you don't belong there, she will call the bouncer and have you removed. She doesn't do it herself – certainly not. Her role is to identify undesirables, not to show them to the door. And it's the same with antibodies: They identify invaders, and let other players do the dirty work.

In developed countries, the invaders we encounter most frequently are bacteria and viruses. Antibodies can bind to both types of invaders and tag them for destruction.

Immunologists like to say that antibodies can **opsonize** these invaders. This term comes from a German word that means "to prepare for eating." I like to equate opsonize with "decorate," because I picture these bacteria and viruses with antibodies hanging all over them, decorating their surfaces. Anyway, when antibodies opsonize bacteria or viruses, they do so by binding to the invader with their Fab regions, leaving their Fc tails available to bind to Fc receptors on the surface of cells such as macrophages. Using this strategy, antibodies can form a bridge between the invader and the phagocyte, bringing the invader in close, and preparing it for phagocytosis.

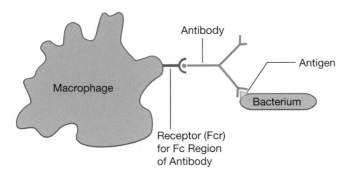

In fact, it's even better than this. When a phagocyte's Fc receptors bind to antibodies that are opsonizing an invader, the appetite of the phagocyte increases, making it even more phagocytic. Macrophages have proteins on their surface that can bind directly to many common invaders. However, the ability of antibodies to form a bridge between a macrophage and an invader allows a macrophage to increase its catalog of enemies to include any invader to which an antibody can bind, common or uncommon. In effect, antibodies focus a macrophage's attention on invaders, some of which (the uncommon ones) a macrophage would otherwise ignore.

During a viral attack, antibodies can do something else that is very important. Viruses enter our cells by binding to certain receptor molecules on a cell's surface. Of course these receptors are not placed there for the convenience of the virus. They are normal receptors, like the Fc receptor, that have quite legitimate functions, but which the virus has learned to use to its own advantage. Once it has bound to these receptors and entered a cell, a virus then uses the cell's machinery to make many copies of itself. These newly made viruses burst out of the cell, sometimes killing it, and go on to infect neighboring cells. Now for the neat part: Antibodies can actually bind to a virus while it is still outside of a cell, and can keep the virus either from entering the cell or from reproducing

once it has entered. Antibodies with these properties are called **neutralizing antibodies**. For example, some neutralizing antibodies can prevent a virus from "docking" on the surface of a cell by binding to the part of the virus that normally would plug into the cellular receptor. When this happens, the virus is "hung out to dry," opsonized and ready to be eaten by phagocytes!

T cells

Although antibodies can tag viruses for phagocytic ingestion, and can help keep viruses from infecting cells, there is a flaw in the antibody defense against viruses: Once a virus gets into a cell, antibodies can't get to it, so the virus is safe to make thousands of copies of itself. Mother Nature recognized this problem, and to deal with it, she invented the famous **killer T cell**, another member of the adaptive immune system team.

The importance of T cells is suggested by the fact that an adult human has about 300 billion of them. T cells are very similar to B cells in appearance. In fact, under an ordinary microscope, an immunologist can't tell them apart. Like B cells, T cells are produced in the bone marrow, and on their surface they display antibody-like molecules called **T cell receptors (TCRs)**. Like the B cell's receptors (the antibody molecules attached to its surface), TCRs also are made by a mix-and-match, modular design strategy. As a result, TCRs are about as diverse as BCRs. T cells also obey the principle of clonal selection: When a T cell's receptors bind to their cognate antigen, the T cell proliferates to build up a clone of T cells with the same specificity. This proliferation stage takes about a week to complete, so like the antibody response, the T cell response is slow and specific.

Although they are similar in many ways, there are also important differences between B cells and T cells. Whereas B cells mature in the bone marrow, T cells mature in the thymus (that's why they're called "T" cells). Further, although B cells make antibodies that can recognize any organic molecule, T cells specialize in recognizing protein antigens. In addition, a B cell can secrete its receptors in the form of antibodies, but a T cell's receptors remain tightly glued to its surface. Perhaps most importantly, a B cell can recognize an antigen "by itself," whereas a T cell, like an old English gentleman, will only recognize an antigen if it is "properly presented" by another cell. I'll explain what that means in a bit.

There are actually three main types of T cells: **killer T cells** (frequently called **cytotoxic lymphocytes** or **CTLs**), helper T cells, and regulatory T cells. The killer T cell is a potent weapon that can destroy virus-infected cells. Indeed, by recognizing and killing these cells, the CTL solves the "hiding virus" problem – the flaw I mentioned in the antibody defense against viruses. The way a killer T cell destroys virus-infected cells is by making contact with its target and then triggering the cell to commit suicide! This "assisted suicide" is a great way to deal with viruses that have infected cells – because when a virus-infected cell dies, the viruses within the cell die also.

The second type of T cell is the **helper T cell (Th cell)**. As you will see, this cell serves as the quarterback of the immune system team. It directs the action by secreting chemical messengers (cytokines) that have dramatic effects on other immune system cells. These cytokines have names like interleukin 2 (IL-2) and interferon gamma (IFN-γ), and we will discuss what they do in later lectures. For now, it is only important to realize that helper T cells are basically cytokine factories.

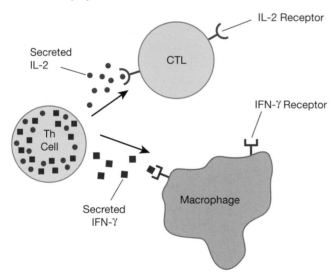

The third type of T cell, the **regulatory T cell (Treg)**, is still somewhat mysterious. The role of regulatory T cells is to help keep the immune system from overreacting – although the details of how this is accomplished are not fully understood.

Antigen presentation

One thing I need to clear up is exactly how antigen is presented to T cells. It turns out that special proteins called **major histocompatibility complex (MHC)** proteins actually do the "presenting," and that T cells use their receptors to "view" this presented antigen. As you may know, "histo" means tissue, and these major histocompatibility proteins, in addition to being presentation molecules, also are involved in the rejection of transplanted organs. In fact,

when you hear that someone is waiting for a "matched" kidney, it's the MHC molecules of the donor and the recipient that the transplant surgeon is trying to match.

There are two types of MHC molecules, called class I and class II. **Class I MHC molecules** are found in varying amounts on the surface of most cells in the body. Class I MHC molecules function as "billboards" which inform killer T cells about what is going on inside these cells. For example, when a human cell is infected by a virus, fragments of viral proteins called **peptides** are loaded onto class I MHC molecules, and transported to the surface of the infected cell. By inspecting these protein fragments displayed by class I MHC molecules, killer T cells can use their receptors to "look into" the cell to discover that it has been infected and that it should be destroyed.

Class II MHC molecules also function as billboards, but this display is intended for the enlightenment of helper T cells. Only certain cells in the body make class II MHC molecules, and these are called **antigen presenting cells (APCs)**. Macrophages, for example, are excellent antigen presenting cells. During a bacterial infection, a macrophage will "eat" bacteria, and will load fragments of ingested bacterial proteins onto class II MHC molecules for display on the surface of the macrophage. Then, using their T cell receptors, helper T cells can scan the macrophage's class II MHC billboards for news of the bacterial infection. So class I MHC molecules alert killer T cells when something isn't right <u>inside</u> a cell, and class II MHC molecules displayed on APCs inform helper T cells that problems exist <u>outside</u> of cells.

Although a class I MHC molecule is made up of one long chain (the heavy chain) plus a short chain (**β2-microglobulin**), and a class II MHC molecule has two long chains (α and β), you'll notice that these molecules are rather similar in appearance.

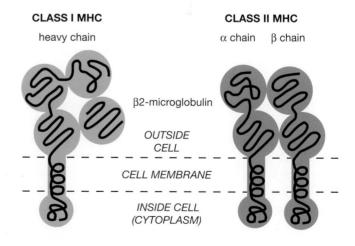

Okay, I know it's hard to visualize the real shapes of molecules from drawings like this, so I thought I'd show you a few pictures that may make this more real. Here's what an empty MHC molecule might look like from the viewpoint of the T cell receptor. Right away you see the groove into which the protein fragment would fit.

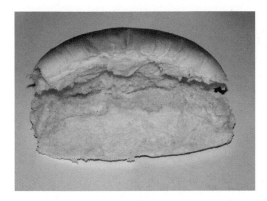

Next, let's look at a fully-loaded, class I molecule.

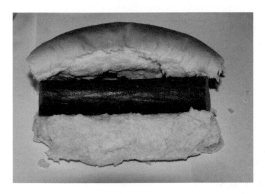

I can tell it's a class I MHC molecule because the peptide is contained nicely within the groove. It turns out that the ends of the groove of a class I molecule are closed, so a protein fragment must be about nine amino acids in length to fit in properly. Class II MHC molecules are slightly different.

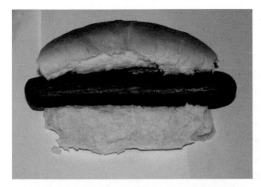

Here you see that the peptide overflows the groove. This works fine for class II, because the ends of the groove are open, so protein fragments as large as about 20 amino acids fit nicely.

So MHC molecules resemble buns, and the protein fragments they present resemble wieners. And if you imagine that the cells in our bodies have hot dogs on their surfaces, you won't be far wrong about antigen presentation. That's certainly the way I picture it!

Activation of the adaptive immune system

Because B and T cells are such potent weapons, Mother Nature put into place the requirement that cells of the adaptive immune system must be activated before they can function. Collectively, B and T cells are called **lymphocytes**, and how they are activated is one of the key issues in immunology. To introduce this concept, I will sketch how helper T cells are activated.

The first step in the activation of a helper T cell is recognition of its cognate antigen (e.g., a fragment of a bacterial protein) displayed by class II MHC molecules on the surface of an antigen presenting cell. But seeing its cognate antigen on that billboard isn't enough – a second signal or "key" also is required for activation. This second signal is non-specific (it's the same for any antigen), and it involves a protein (B7 in this drawing) on the surface of an antigen presenting cell that plugs into its receptor (CD28 in this drawing) on the surface of the helper T cell.

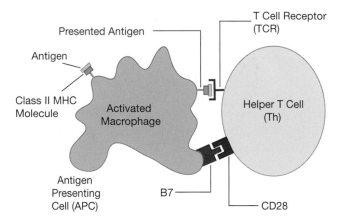

You see an example of this kind of two-key system when you visit your safe deposit box. You bring with you a key that is specific for your box – it won't fit any other. The bank teller provides a second, non-specific key that will fit all the boxes. Only when both keys are inserted into the locks on your box can it be opened. Your specific key alone won't do it, and the teller's non-specific key alone won't either. You need both. Now, why do you suppose helper T cells and other cells of the adaptive immune system require two keys for activation? For safety, of course – just like your bank box. These cells are powerful weapons that must only be activated at the appropriate time and place.

Once a helper T cell has been activated by this two-key system, it proliferates to build up a clone composed of many helper T cells whose receptors recognize the same antigen. These helper cells then mature into cells that can produce the cytokines needed to direct the activities of the immune system. B cells and killer T cells also require two-key systems for their activation, and we'll talk about them in another lecture.

The secondary lymphoid organs

If you've been thinking about how the adaptive immune system might get turned on during an attack, you've probably begun to wonder whether this could ever happen. After all, there are only between 100 and 1000 T cells that will have TCRs specific for a given invader, and for these T cells to be activated, they must come in contact with an antigen presenting cell that has "seen" that invader. Given that these T cells and APCs are spread all over the body, it would not seem very likely that this would happen before an invasion got completely out of hand. Fortunately, to make this system work with reasonable probability, Mother Nature invented the **secondary lymphoid organs**, the best known of which is the **lymph node**. You may not be familiar with the **lymphatic system**, so I'd better say a few words about it.

In your home, you have two plumbing systems. The first supplies the water that comes out of your faucets. This is a pressurized system, with the pressure being provided by a pump. You have another plumbing system that includes the drains in your sinks, showers, and toilets. This second system is not under pressure – the water just flows down the drain and out into the sewer. The two systems are connected in the sense that eventually the wastewater is recycled and used again.

The plumbing in a human is very much like this. We have a pressurized system (the cardiovascular system) in which blood is pumped around the body by the heart. Everybody knows about this one. But we also have another plumbing system: the lymphatic system. This system is not under pressure, and it drains the fluid (lymph) that leaks out of our blood vessels into our tissues. Without this system, our tissues would fill up with fluid and we'd look like the Pillsbury Doughboy. Fortunately, lymph is collected from the tissues of our lower body into lymphatic vessels, and is transported by these vessels, under the influence of muscular contraction, through a series

of one-way valves to the upper torso. This lymph, plus lymph from the left side of the upper torso, is collected into the thoracic duct and emptied into the left subclavian vein to be recycled back into the blood. Likewise, lymph from the right side of the upper body is collected into the right lymphatic duct and is emptied into the right subclavian vein. From this diagram, you can see that as the lymph winds its way back to be reunited with the blood, it passes through a series of way stations – the lymph nodes.

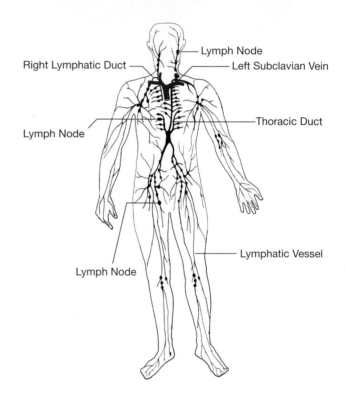

In a human, there are about 500 lymph nodes that range in size from very small to almost as big as a Brussels sprout. Most are arrayed in "chains" that are connected by lymphatic vessels. Invaders such as bacteria and viruses are carried by the lymph to nearby nodes, and antigen presenting cells that have picked up foreign antigens in the tissues travel to lymph nodes to present their cargo. Meanwhile, B cells and T cells circulate from node to node, looking for the antigens for which they are "fated." So lymph nodes really function as "dating bars" – places where T cells, B cells, APCs, and antigen all gather for the purpose of communication and activation. Bringing these cells and antigens together within the small volume of a lymph node greatly increases the probability that they will interact and efficiently activate the adaptive immune system.

Immunological memory

After B and T cells have been activated, have proliferated to build up clones of cells with identical antigen specificities, and have vanquished the enemy, most of them die off. This is a good idea, because we wouldn't want our immune systems to fill up with old B and T cells. On the other hand, it would be nice if some of these experienced B and T cells would stick around, just in case we are exposed to the same invaders again. That way, the adaptive immune system wouldn't have to start from scratch. And that's just the way it works. These "leftover" B and T cells are called **memory cells**, and in addition to being more numerous than the original, inexperienced B and T cells, memory cells are easier to activate. As a result of this immunological memory, during a second attack, the adaptive system usually can spring into action so quickly that you never even experience any symptoms.

Tolerance of self

As I mentioned earlier, B cell receptors and T cell receptors are so diverse that they should be able to recognize any potential invader. However, this diversity raises a problem: If B and T cell receptors are this diverse, many of them are certain to recognize our own "self" molecules (e.g., the molecules that make up our cells, or proteins like insulin that circulate in our blood). If this were to happen, our adaptive immune system might attack our own bodies, and we could die from autoimmune disease. Fortunately, Mother Nature has devised ways to educate B cells and T cells to discriminate between ourselves and dangerous invaders. Although the mechanisms involved in teaching B and T cells to be tolerant of our self antigens still are not completely understood, the education which B and T cells receive is sufficiently rigorous that autoimmune disease is relatively rare.

A COMPARISON OF THE INNATE AND ADAPTIVE IMMUNE SYSTEMS

Now that you have met some of the main players, I want to emphasize the differences between the innate and adaptive immune system "teams." Understanding how they differ is crucial to understanding how the immune system works.

Imagine that you are in the middle of town and someone steals your shoes. You look around for a store where you can buy another pair, and the first store you see is called Charlie's Custom Shoes. This store has shoes of every style, color, and size, and the salesperson is able to fit you in exactly the shoes you need. However, when it comes time to pay, you are told that you must wait a week or two to get your shoes – they will have to be custom-made for you, and that will take a while. But you need shoes right now! You are barefoot, and you must have something to put on your feet until those custom shoes arrive. So they send you across the street to Freddie's Fast Fit – a store that only carries a few styles and sizes. Freddie's wouldn't be able to fit Shaquille O'Neal, but this store does stock shoes in the common sizes that fit most people. Consequently, you can buy a pair of shoes from Freddie's that will tide you over until your custom shoes are made for you.

This is very similar to the way the innate and adaptive immune systems work. The players of the innate system (like the macrophage) are already in place, and are ready to defend against a relatively small attack by invaders we are likely to meet on a day-to-day basis. Indeed, in many instances, the innate system is so effective and so fast that the adaptive immune system never even kicks in. In other cases, the innate system may be insufficient to deal with an invasion, and the adaptive system will need to be mobilized. This takes time, however, because the B and T cells of the adaptive system must be custom-made through the process of clonal selection and proliferation. Consequently, while these "designer cells" are being produced, the innate immune system must do its best to hold the invaders at bay.

THE INNATE SYSTEM RULES!

Immunologists used to believe that the only function of the innate system was to provide a rapid defense which would deal with invaders while the adaptive immune system was getting cranked up. However, it is now clear that the innate system does much more than that.

The adaptive immune system's antigen receptors (BCRs and TCRs) are so diverse that they can probably recognize any protein molecule in the universe. However, the adaptive system is clueless as to which of these molecules is dangerous and which is not. So how does the adaptive system distinguish friend from foe? The answer is that it relies on the judgment of the innate system.

In contrast to the antigen receptors of the adaptive immune system, which are totally "unfocused," the receptors of the innate system are precisely tuned to detect the presence of the common pathogens (disease-causing agents) we encounter in daily life – viruses, bacteria, fungi, and parasites. In addition, the innate system has receptors that can detect when "uncommon" pathogens kill human cells. Consequently, it is the innate system which is responsible for evaluating the danger and for activating the adaptive immune system. In a real sense, the innate system gives "permission" to the adaptive system to respond to an invasion. But it's even better than that, because the innate system does more than just turn the adaptive system on. The innate system actually integrates all the information it collects about an invader, and formulates a plan of action. This "game plan," which the innate system delivers to the adaptive immune system, tells which weapons must be mobilized (e.g., B cells or killer T cells) and exactly where in the body these weapons should be deployed. So if we think of the helper T cell as the quarterback of the adaptive immune system team, we should consider the innate immune system to be the "coach" – for it is the innate system which "scouts" the opponents, designs the game plan, and sends in the plays for the quarterback to call.

EPILOGUE

We have come to the end of our turbo overview of the immune system, and by now you should have a rough idea of how the system works. In the next nine lectures, we will focus more sharply on the individual players of the innate and adaptive system teams, paying special attention to how and where these players interact with each other to make the system function efficiently.

LECTURE 2

The Innate Immune System

HEADS UP!

The innate immune system is a "hard-wired" defense that has evolved over millions of years to recognize pathogens that commonly infect humans. The innate system team includes the complement system of proteins, the professional phagocytes, and natural killer cells. Before they can fight, these warriors must be activated. Cooperation between innate system players is critical to insure a fast and effective response against "everyday" invaders.

INTRODUCTION

For years, immunologists didn't pay much attention to the innate system – because the adaptive system seemed more interesting. However, studies of the adaptive immune system have led to a new appreciation of the role that the innate system plays, not only as a lightning-fast, second line of defense (if we count physical barriers as our first defense), but also as an activator and a controller of the adaptive immune system.

It's easy to understand the importance of the innate system's quick response to common invaders if you think about what could happen in an uncontrolled bacterial infection. Imagine that the splinter from your hot tub deck introduced just one bacterium into your tissues. As you know, bacteria multiply very quickly. In fact, a single bacterium doubling in number every 30 minutes could give rise to roughly 100 trillion bacteria in one day. If you've ever worked with bacterial cultures, you know that a 1-liter culture containing one trillion bacteria is so dense you can't see through it. So, a single bacterium proliferating for one day could yield a dense culture of about 100 liters. Now remember that your total blood volume is only about 5 liters, and you can appreciate what an unchecked bacterial infection could do to a human! Without the quick-acting innate immune system to defend us, we would clearly be in big trouble.

The weapons of the innate immune system include the complement proteins, the professional phagocytes, and natural killer cells. We'll begin our discussion with my favorite: the complement system.

THE COMPLEMENT SYSTEM

The complement system is composed of about 20 different proteins that work together to destroy invaders and to signal other immune system players that the attack is on. The complement system is very old. Even sea urchins, which evolved about 700 million years ago, have a complement system. In humans, complement proteins start being made during the first trimester of fetal development, so it's clear that Mother Nature wants this important system to be ready to go well before a child is born. Indeed, those rare humans born with a defect in one of the major complement proteins usually do not live long before succumbing to infection.

When I first read about the complement system, I thought it was way too complicated to even bother understanding. But as I studied it further, I began to realize that it is really quite simple and elegant. As with just about everything else in the immune defense, the complement system must be activated before it can function, and there are three ways this can happen. The first, the so-called "classical" pathway, depends on antibodies for activation, so we'll save that for a later lecture. Because the way the complement system functions is independent of how it is activated, you won't miss much by waiting to hear about the antibody-dependent pathway of activation.

The alternative pathway

The second way the complement system can be activated is called the **alternative pathway**. Although in evolutionary terms, the alternative pathway certainly evolved before the classical pathway, immunologists call the antibody-dependent activation "classical" simply because it happened to be discovered first.

The proteins that make up the complement system are produced mainly by the liver, and are present at high concentrations in blood and tissues. The most abundant complement protein is called C3, and in the human body C3 molecules are continually being broken into two smaller proteins. One of the protein fragments created by this "spontaneous" cleavage, C3b, is very reactive, and can bind to either of two common chemical groups (amino or hydroxyl groups). Because many of the proteins and carbohydrates that make up the surfaces of invaders (e.g., bacterial cells) have amino or hydroxyl groups, there are lots of targets for these little C3b "grenades."

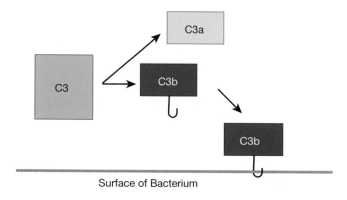

Surface of Bacterium

If C3b doesn't find one of these chemical groups to react with within about 60 microseconds, it is neutralized by binding to a water molecule, and the game is over. This means the spontaneously clipped C3 molecule has to be right up close to the surface of the invading cell in order for the complement cascade to continue. Once C3b is stabilized by reacting with a molecule on the cell surface, another complement protein, B, binds to C3b, and complement protein D comes along and clips off part of B to yield C3bBb.

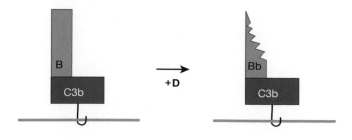

Once a bacterium has this C3bBb molecule glued to its surface, the fun really begins, because C3bBb acts like a "chain saw" that can cut other C3 proteins and convert them to C3b. Consequently, C3 molecules that are in the neighborhood don't have to wait for spontaneous clipping events to convert them to C3b – the C3bBb molecule (called a **convertase**) can do the job very efficiently. And once another C3 molecule has been clipped, it too can bind to an amino or hydroxyl group on the surface of the bacterium.

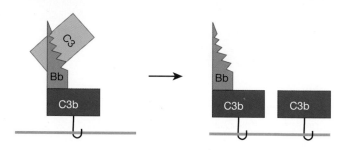

This process can continue, and pretty soon there will be lots of C3b molecules attached to the surface of the target bacterium – and each of them can form a C3bBb convertase – which can then cut even more C3 molecules. All this attaching and cutting sets up a positive feedback loop, and the whole process just snowballs.

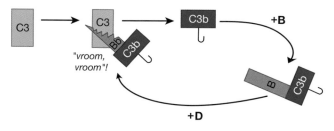

Once C3b is bound to the surface of a bacterium, the complement cascade can proceed further. The C3bBb chain saw can bind to another molecule of C3b, and together they can clip a complement protein, C5, into two pieces. One of these pieces, C5b, can then combine with other complement proteins (C6, C7, C8, and C9) to make a **membrane attack complex (MAC)**. To form this structure, C5b, C6, C7, and C8 form a "stalk" that anchors the complex in the bacterial cell membrane. Then C9 proteins are added to make a channel that opens up a hole in the surface of the bacterium. And once a bacterium has a hole in its surface, it's toast!

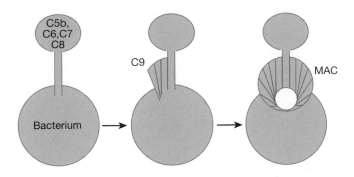

I have used a bacterium as our "model pathogen," but the complement system also can defend against other invaders such as parasites and even some viruses. Now, you may be thinking: With these grenades going off all over the place, why doesn't the complement system form membrane attack complexes on the surface of our own cells? The answer is that human cells are equipped with many safeguards that keep this from happening. In fact, Mother Nature was so worried about the complement system reacting inappropriately that she devoted about as many proteins to controlling the complement system as there are proteins in the system itself! For instance, the complement fragment, C3b, can be clipped to an inactive form by proteins in the blood, and this clipping is accelerated by an enzyme (MCP) that is present on the surface of human cells. There is also a protein on human cells called decay accelerating factor (DAF) which accelerates the destruction of the convertase, C3bBb, by other blood proteins. This can keep the positive feedback loop from getting started. And yet another cell-surface protein, CD59 (also called protectin), prevents the incorporation of C9 molecules into nascent MACs.

An interesting story illustrates why these safeguards are so important. Transplant surgeons don't have enough human organs to satisfy the demand for transplantation, so they are considering using organs from animals. One of the hot candidates for an organ donor is the pig, because pigs are cheap to raise and some of their organs are about the same size as those of humans. As a warm-up for human transplantation, surgeons decided to transplant a pig organ into a baboon. This experiment was not a big success! Almost immediately, the baboon's immune system began to attack the organ, and within minutes the transplanted organ was a bloody pulp. The culprit? The complement system. It turns out that the pig versions of DAF and CD59 don't work to control primate complement, so the unprotected pig organ was vulnerable to attack by the baboon's complement system.

This story highlights two important features of the complement system. First, **the complement system works very fast.** Complement proteins are present at high concentrations in blood and in tissues, and they are ready to go against any invader that has a surface with a spare hydroxyl or amino group. A second characteristic of this system is that **if a cell surface is not protected, it will be attacked by complement. In fact, the picture you should have is that the complement system is continually dropping these little grenades, and any unprotected surface will be a target. In this system, the default option is death!**

The lectin activation pathway

In addition to the classical (antibody-dependent) and alternative (antibody-independent) pathways of complement activation, there is a third pathway that may be the most important activation pathway of all: the **lectin activation pathway**. The central player in this pathway is a protein that is produced mainly in the liver, and which is present in moderate concentrations in the blood and tissues. This protein is called **mannose-binding lectin (MBL)**. A lectin is a protein that is able to bind to a carbohydrate molecule, and mannose is a carbohydrate molecule found on the surface of many common pathogens. For example, MBL has been shown to bind to yeasts such as *Candida albicans*; to viruses such as HIV-1 and influenza A; to many bacteria, including *Salmonella* and *Streptococcus*; and to parasites such as *Leishmania*. In contrast, MBL does not bind to the carbohydrates found on healthy human cells and tissues. This is an example of an important strategy employed by the innate system: **The innate system mainly focuses on patterns of carbohydrates and fats that are found on the surface of common pathogens, but not on the surface of human cells.**

The way mannose-binding lectin works to activate the complement system is very simple. In the blood, MBL binds to another protein called MASP. Then, when the mannose-binding lectin grabs its target (mannose on the surface of a bacterium, for example), the MASP protein functions like a convertase to clip C3 complement proteins to make C3b. Because C3 is so abundant in the blood, this happens very efficiently. The C3b fragments can then bind to the surface of the bacterium, and the complement chain reaction we just discussed will be off and running. So, **whereas the alternative activation pathway is spontaneous, and can be visualized as grenades going off randomly here and there to destroy any unprotected surface, lectin activation can be thought of as "smart bombs" that are targeted by mannose-binding lectins.**

Other complement system functions

In addition to building membrane attack complexes, the complement system has two other important functions. When C3b has attached itself to the surface of an invader, it can be clipped by a serum protein to produce a smaller fragment, iC3b. The "i" prefix denotes that this cleaved protein is now inactive for making MACs. However, it is still glued to the invader, and it can prepare the invader for phagocytosis (i.e., can opsonize it) in much the same way that invaders can be opsonized by antibodies. On the surface of phagocytes (e.g., macrophages) are receptors that can bind to iC3b, and the binding of iC3b-opsonized invaders facilitates phagocytosis. Many invaders have surfaces that are rather "slimy," making them difficult for macrophages to grasp. However, when these slippery invaders are coated with complement fragments, phagocytes can get a better grip. Thus, **a second function of complement is to decorate the surfaces of invaders, thereby acting like a "poor man's antibody" in opsonization.**

The complement system has a third important function: **Fragments of complement proteins can serve as** **chemoattractants** — **chemicals that recruit other immune system players to the battle site.** For example, **C3a** and **C5a** are the pieces of C3 and C5 that are clipped off when C3b and C5b are made (let nothing be wasted!). These fragments don't bind to the surface of invaders. Rather, they are set free in the tissues where they function as chemoattractants. C5a is an especially powerful chemoattractant for macrophages, and can activate them so that they become more potent killers. Interestingly, these fragments, C3a and C5a, are called **anaphylatoxins**, because they can contribute to anaphylactic shock – something we will talk about in another lecture.

So the complement system is quite multifunctional: **It can destroy invaders by building membrane attack complexes; it can tag intruders for destruction by phagocytes; it can alert other cells that we are being attacked, and direct them to the battle scene; and it can help activate them. Most importantly, it can do all these things very fast.**

THE PROFESSIONAL PHAGOCYTES

Professional phagocytes comprise the second arm of the innate system. These cells are called "professional" because they make their living mainly by eating (phagocytosis). The most important professional phagocytes are the macrophages and the neutrophils.

Macrophages – immune system sentinels

Macrophages are found under your skin, where they provide protection against invaders which penetrate this barrier and gain entry into your tissues (e.g., as the result of a wound or a burn). Macrophages also are present in your lungs, where they defend against inhaled microbes. Still other macrophages reside in the tissues that surround your intestines. There they lie in wait for microbial invaders you have ingested, which have escaped the confines of your intestines, and which have entered your tissues. Indeed, macrophages are sentinel cells that can be found just below the surface in all areas of your body which are exposed to the outside world – areas that are prime targets for microbial infection.

Macrophages can exist in three stages of readiness. In tissues, they are usually found just lounging and slowly proliferating. In this "resting" state, they function primarily as garbage collectors, taking sips of whatever is around them, and keeping our tissues free of debris. About one million cells die per second in an adult human, so macrophages have a lot of tidying up to do. Dying cells give off "find me" signals that attract macrophages, bringing them close enough to recognize "eat me" signals displayed on the surface of cells when they die.

While resting, macrophages express very few class II MHC molecules on their surface, so they aren't much good at presenting antigen to helper T cells. This makes sense. Why would they want to present garbage anyway? For the average macrophage, life is pretty boring. They live for months in tissues and just collect garbage.

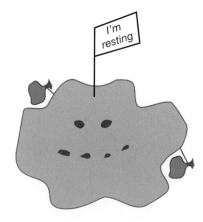

Every once in a while, however, some of these resting macrophages receive signals which alert them that the barrier defense has been penetrated, and that there are intruders in the area. When this happens, they become activated (or "primed," as immunologists usually say). In this state, macrophages take larger gulps and upregulate expression of class II MHC molecules. Now a macrophage can function as an antigen presenting cell, and when it engulfs invaders, it can use its class II MHC molecules to display fragments of the invaders' proteins for helper T cells to see. Although a number of different signals can prime a resting macrophage, the best studied is an intercellular communication molecule (cytokine) called **interferon gamma (IFN-γ)**. This cytokine is produced mainly by helper T cells and natural killer cells.

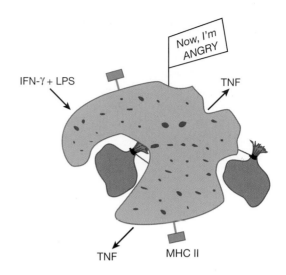

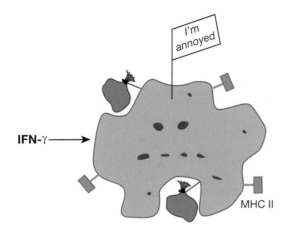

In the primed state, macrophages are good antigen presenters and reasonably good killers. However, there is an even higher state of readiness, "hyperactivation," which they can attain if they receive a direct signal from an invader. Such a signal can be conveyed, for example, by a molecule called **lipopolysaccharide (LPS)**. LPS, a component of the outer cell membrane of Gram-negative bacteria such as *Escherichia coli*, can be shed by these bacteria, and can bind to receptors on the surface of primed macrophages. Macrophages also have receptors for mannose. When receptors on the surface of the macrophage bind to "danger signals" such as LPS or mannose, the macrophage knows for sure that there has been an invasion. Faced with this realization, the macrophage stops proliferating, and focuses its attention on killing. In the hyperactive state, macrophages grow larger and increase their rate of phagocytosis. In fact, they become so large and phagocytic that they can ingest invaders that are as big as unicellular parasites. Hyperactivated macrophages also produce and secrete another cytokine, **tumor necrosis factor (TNF)**. This cytokine can kill tumor cells and virus-infected cells, and can help activate other immune system warriors.

Inside a hyperactivated macrophage, the number of lysosomes increases, so that the destruction of ingested invaders becomes more efficient. In addition, hyperactivated macrophages increase production of reactive oxygen molecules such as hydrogen peroxide. You know what peroxide can do to hair, so you can imagine what it might do to a bacterium! Finally, when hyperactivated, a macrophage can dump the contents of its lysosomes onto multicellular parasites, enabling it to destroy invaders that are too large to "eat." Yes, a hyperactivated macrophage is a killing machine!

So a macrophage is a very versatile cell. It can function as a garbage collector, as an antigen presenting cell, or as a vicious killer – depending on its activation level. However, you shouldn't get the impression that macrophages have three "gears." Nothing in immunology has gears, and the activation state of a macrophage is a continuum that really depends on the type and the strength of the activation signals it receives.

Usually, macrophages are able to deal with small attacks. However, when invaders are numerous, macrophages risk being overpowered, and in these cases, macrophages call for backup. The most common reinforcement for battling macrophages is a cell called a **neutrophil**. Indeed, although the macrophage is unmatched in versatility, the most important of the professional phagocytes is probably the neutrophil.

Neutrophils – the immune system's foot soldiers

All of our cells receive their nutrients from the blood, and consequently no cell is more than about the thickness of a fingernail from a blood vessel. If a cell is farther away than that, it will die of starvation. Because our tissues are laced with blood vessels, blood is the perfect vehicle for bringing reinforcements to parts of the body that are under attack. And circulating through our veins and arteries are about 20 billion neutrophils. In contrast to macrophages, which can be thought of as sentinels, neutrophils are more like "foot soldiers." Their job is to "kill things and break stuff," and they are really good at this.

Neutrophils live a very short time. In fact, they come out of the bone marrow programmed to die in an average of about five days. In contrast to macrophages, neutrophils are not antigen presenting cells. They are professional killers which are "on call" from the blood.

Once they have been summoned, it only takes neutrophils about half an hour to exit the blood and become fully activated. In this state, neutrophils are incredibly phagocytic, and once their prey has been taken inside, a whole battery of powerful chemicals awaits the unlucky "guest." Neutrophils also produce battle cytokines (e.g., TNF) that can alert other immune system cells. And most importantly, activated neutrophils give off destructive chemicals which are pre-made and stored inside the neutrophil until needed. These chemicals can turn tissues into a "toxic soup" that is lethal to invading microbes. Indeed, neutrophils are unique in that they are the only immune system cells that are "licensed" to liquify both cells and connective tissue.

My friend Dan Tenen studies neutrophils. Another friend, Linda Clayton, who experiments with T cells, likes to kid him by asking, "Why do you bother studying neutrophils, Dan? All they do is dive into pus and die!" She's right, of course. Pus is mainly dead neutrophils. However, Dan reminds her that humans can live for long periods without her fancy T cells, but without his neutrophils they will succumb to infection and die within a matter of days.

Now, why do you think Mother Nature set things up so that macrophages are very long lived, yet neutrophils live only a few days? Doesn't that seem wasteful? Why not let neutrophils enjoy a long life, just like macrophages? That's right! It would be too dangerous. Neutrophils come out of blood vessels ready to kill, and in the course of this killing, there is always damage to normal tissues. So to limit collateral damage, neutrophils are programmed to be short lived. If the battle requires additional neutrophils, more can be recruited from the blood – there are plenty of them there. Indeed, neutrophils represent about 70% of the circulating white blood cells. In contrast, because macrophages act as sentinels that watch for invaders and signal the attack, it makes sense that macrophages should live a long time out in the tissues.

How neutrophils exit the blood

You may be wondering: If neutrophils are all that dangerous, how do they know when to leave the blood stream and where to go? It certainly wouldn't do to have neutrophils leave the blood and become activated just any old place. No indeed, and the way this works is very clever. Inside blood vessels, neutrophils exist in an inactive state, and they are swept along by the blood at high speed: about 1000 microns per second. If you're the size of a neutrophil, that's really fast.

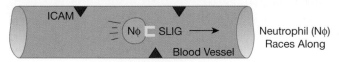

NORMAL TISSUE

In this sketch, you will notice that there is a protein, intercellular adhesion molecule (ICAM), which is expressed on the surface of the endothelial cells that line blood vessels. There is also another adhesion molecule called selectin ligand (SLIG) that is expressed on the surface of neutrophils. As you can see, however, these two adhesion molecules are not "partners," so they don't bind to each other, and the neutrophil is free to zip along with the flowing blood.

Now imagine that you get a splinter in your big toe, and that the bacteria on the splinter activate macrophages which are standing guard in the tissues of your foot. These activated macrophages give off cytokines, **interleukin 1 (IL-1)** and TNF, which signal that an invasion has begun. When endothelial cells that line nearby blood vessels receive these alarm signals, they begin to express a new protein on their surface called selectin (SEL). It normally takes about 6 hours for this protein to be made and transported to the surface of endothelial cells. Selectin is the adhesion partner for selectin ligand, so when selectin is expressed on the endothelial cell surface, it functions like Velcro to grab neutrophils as they fly by. However, this interaction between selectin and its ligand is only strong enough to cause neutrophils to slow down and roll along the inner surface of the blood vessel.

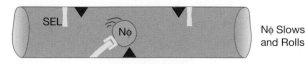

**INFLAMED TISSUE
IL-1 AND TNF**

As a neutrophil rolls, it "sniffs." What it's sniffing for is a signal that there is a battle (an inflammatory reaction) going on in the tissues. The complement fragment C5a and LPS are two of the inflammatory signals that a neutrophil recognizes. When it receives such signals, the neutrophil rushes a new protein called integrin (INT) to its surface. This quick reaction is important, because the neutrophil hasn't stopped – it's still rolling along. If it rolls too far, it will leave the region where selectin is expressed, and will then start to zoom along again at "blood speed." To make rapid surface expression of integrin possible, a lot of this protein is made in advance by the neutrophil and is stored inside the cell until needed.

When integrin appears on the neutrophil's surface, it interacts with its binding partner ICAM, which always is expressed on the surface of endothelial cells. This interaction is very strong, and it causes the neutrophil to stop rolling.

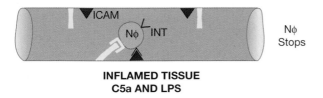

INFLAMED TISSUE
C5a AND LPS

Once a neutrophil has stopped, it can be encouraged by chemoattractants to pry apart the endothelial cells that line the blood vessels, exit into the tissues, and migrate to the site of inflammation. These chemoattractants include the complement fragment C5a and fragments of bacterial proteins called **f-met peptides**. Bacterial proteins begin with a special initiator amino acid called formyl methionine (f-met). In human cells, only mitochondria produce proteins with this initiator, so less than 0.1% of all human proteins contain this amino acid. Bacteria secrete f-met peptides, and macrophages burp them up as they ingest bacteria. Consequently, C5a and f-met peptides function as "find me" signals to help phagocytes locate invaders which have been identified as dangerous by the innate system. And as they travel through the tissues, neutrophils can be activated by cytokines such as TNF. As a result, they arrive at the battle scene ready to kill.

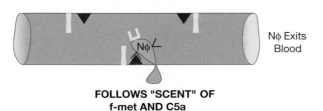

FOLLOWS "SCENT" OF
f-met AND C5a

Neutrophil logic

This system – involving selectin–selectin ligand binding to make the neutrophil roll, integrin–ICAM interactions to stop the neutrophil, and chemoattractants and their receptors to encourage the neutrophil to exit from the blood – may seem overly complicated. Wouldn't it be simpler just to have one pair of adhesion molecules (say, selectin and its ligand) do all three things? Yes, it would be simpler, but it would also be very dangerous. In a human there are about 100 billion endothelial cells. Suppose one of them gets a little crazy and begins to express a lot of selectin on its surface. If selectin binding were the only requirement, neutrophils could empty out of the blood into normal tissues where they could do terrible damage. Having three types of molecules which must be expressed before neutrophils can exit the blood and spring into action helps make the system fail-safe.

You remember I mentioned that to completely upregulate expression of that first cellular adhesion molecule, selectin, takes about 6 hours. Doesn't this seem a bit too leisurely? Wouldn't it be better to begin recruiting neutrophils from the blood just as soon as a macrophage senses danger? Not really. Before you start to recruit reinforcements, you want to be sure that the attack is serious. If a macrophage encounters only a few invaders, it can usually handle the situation without help in a short time. In contrast, a major invasion involving many macrophages can go on for days. The sustained expression of alarm cytokines from many macrophages engaged in battle is required to upregulate selectin expression, and this insures that more troops will be summoned only when they really are needed.

Neutrophils are not the only blood cells that need to exit the blood and enter tissues. For example, eosinophils and mast cells, which are involved in protection against parasites, must exit the blood at the site of a parasitic infection. Monocytes, which can mature into tissue macrophages, need to leave the blood stream at appropriate places. And activated B cells and T cells must be dispatched to sites of infection. This whole business is like a postal system in which there are trillions of packages (immune system cells) that must be delivered to the correct destinations. This delivery problem is solved by using the same basic strategy that works so well for neutrophils. The key feature of the immune system's "postal service" is that the Velcro-like molecules which cause the cells to roll and stop are different from cell type to cell type and destination to destination. As a result, these cellular adhesion molecules actually serve as "zip codes" to insure that cells are delivered to the appropriate locations. Indeed, the selectins and their ligands are really families of molecules, and only certain members of the selectin family will pair up with certain members of the selectin ligand family. The same is true of the integrins and their ligands. Because of this two-digit zip code (type of selectin, type of integrin), there are enough "addresses" available to send the many different immune system cells to all the right places. **By equipping immune system cells with different adhesion molecules, and by equipping their intended destinations with the corresponding adhesion partners, Mother Nature makes sure that the different types of immune system cells will roll, stop, and exit the blood exactly where they are needed.**

HOW IMMUNE SYSTEM SENTINELS RECOGNIZE INVADERS

Before immune system cells like macrophages can spring into action, they must first recognize that there has been an invasion. But how do they do this? The answer is that immune system cells come equipped with an array of **pattern-recognition receptors (PRRs)** which are designed to recognize "danger signals" associated with a microbial attack. Some of these receptors detect **pathogen-associated molecular patterns (PAMPs)** that are characteristic of broad classes of invaders. Other PRRs are tuned to recognize **damage-associated molecular patterns (DAMPs)**. These molecules are normally intracellular, but are released by dying cells (e.g., cells killed by viruses). When invaders are detected by PRRs, warrior cells like macrophages are activated, and battle cytokines are produced which alert and activate other immune system cells.

The PRRs about which most is known are the **Toll-like receptors (TLRs)**. So far, 10 human TLRs have been discovered, and different cells express different combinations of these TLRs. Some TLRs are displayed on the cell surface, where they respond to invaders that are outside the cell. For example, one of the external PRRs, **TLR4**, is used by macrophages to sense the presence of LPS – a PAMP which is a component of the cell membranes of some bacteria. TLR4 is anchored in the macrophage's plasma membrane and points outward to sense bacterial invaders in the external environment.

Other PRRs are found inside cells, and these receptors detect invaders that are within these cells. For instance, when invaders are phagocytosed they end up in phago-lysosomes, where eventually they are destroyed. Dur-

ing this destruction, their "coats" are stripped off to reveal what's inside them. Some of the Toll-like receptors (e.g., **TLR7** and **TLR9**) are located in the membranes of phago-lysosomes. These pattern-recognition receptors point inward into the phago-lysosome so that they can alert the cell to the presence of viruses or bacteria that have been phagocytosed. TLR7 detects the single-stranded RNA of viruses such as influenza and HIV-1, whereas TLR9 recognizes the double-stranded DNA of bacteria and herpes simplex virus.

Pattern-recognition receptors have two important properties. First, **PRRs recognize general characteristics of classes of invaders – not just a single invader.** For example, LPS is a component of the cell membrane of many different bacteria, and single-stranded RNA is found in many viruses. Consequently, TLR4 can detect invasions by many different types of bacteria (those with LPS in their cell membrane), and TLR7 can alert cells to attacks by many different viruses (those which carry their genetic information in the form of single-stranded RNA). So in contrast to B cell receptors and T cell receptors, which are specific for each invader, pattern-recognition receptors are "economical" in the sense that each one can identify many different pathogens.

The second important characteristic of the patterns which PRRs recognize is that they represent structural features which are so important to the pathogen that they cannot easily be altered by mutation to avoid detection. For example, TLR4 has evolved to recognize a region of the LPS molecule that is indispensable for constructing bacterial outer membranes. Consequently, a bacterium would be in big trouble if that part of the LPS molecule were mutated to try to evade detection by TLR4.

HOW THE INNATE IMMUNE SYSTEM DEALS WITH VIRUSES

When a virus infects a human cell, it takes over the cell's machinery and uses it to produce many more copies of the virus. Eventually, the newly made viruses burst out of the infected cell, and go on to infect other cells in the neighborhood. We have already discussed some of the weapons the innate system can use to defend against viruses while they are outside of cells. For example, proteins of the complement system can opsonize viruses for phagocytosis by macrophages and neutrophils. In addition, complement proteins can poke holes in enveloped viruses (e.g., HIV-1) by constructing membrane attack complexes on the virus's surface. However, once a virus has entered a cell to begin its reproductive cycle, these weapons are ineffective. Fortunately, there are other innate system weapons which are useful against virus-infected cells.

The interferon system

Although viruses can be tagged by complement proteins and ingested by phagocytes, the innate system weapon that viruses fear most is the **interferon system**. Indeed, every virus has evolved ways to try to fend off the interferon system at least long enough for the virus to reproduce and spread to a new host.

When the pattern-recognition receptors of innate system cells such as macrophages detect a virus attack, the cells produce "warning proteins" called **interferon alpha (IFN-α) and interferon beta (IFN-β)**. These proteins are called **type I interferons** to distinguish them from IFN-γ, mentioned earlier, which is a type II interferon. IFN-α and IFN-β are called interferons because these proteins function to "interfere" with viral reproduction. Although macrophages and other cells can produce type I interferon, by far the "King of Interferon" is the **plasmacytoid dendritic cell (pDC)**. Human pDCs use TLR7 and TLR9 to detect viral RNA and DNA, respectively, and within about 6 hours of activation, pDCs dedicate more than half of their protein-making capacity to making interferon. As a result, a plasmacytoid dendritic cell can make up to 1000 times as much type I interferon per day as any other cell type! Consequently, these "interferon factories" play a critical role in the innate system's defense against viruses. Here's how this works.

Most human cells have receptors on their surface for type I interferons. When the interferons produced by sentinel cells bind to these receptors on nearby cells, those cells are warned that there are viruses in the area, and that they may soon be attacked. As a result of this warning, the alerted cell turns on expression of several hundred genes which encode proteins that can slow viral reproduction, and which can cause the warned cell to commit suicide if it is infected.

The elegant part of the interferon warning system is that **although the binding of interferon to its receptors prepares a cell for a viral attack, that cell continues to do business as usual unless an attack actually occurs. The alerted cell will only commit suicide if it is infected by a virus.** Of course, for the cell, this is an altruistic act – because both the cell and the virus die together. Nevertheless, this "beneficial suicide" does prevent the virus from reproducing and infecting other cells. And if the attack does not come, the warned cell eventually "stands down" from its state of readiness.

Natural killer cells

There is another important player on the innate immune system team which can help defend against a viral infection: the **natural killer (NK) cell**. Indeed, humans with genetic defects which make them deficient in NK cell function have great difficulty controlling herpes virus and human papillomavirus infections.

Natural killer cells mature in the bone marrow and, when they are not responding to an infection, are short-lived with a half life of only about a week. Most NK cells are found in the blood or in the spleen and liver (two organs that store blood), and very few NK cells reside in tissues that are not under attack. So, like neutrophils, natural killer cells are on call. They use the "roll, stop, exit" strategy to leave the blood and enter tissues at sites of infection – and once in the tissues, they proliferate rapidly to build up their numbers.

When they reach the battleground, natural killer cells can play two roles in defending us against infections. First, **NK cells can give off cytokines such as IFN-γ that help with the defense.** Like macrophages, NK cells

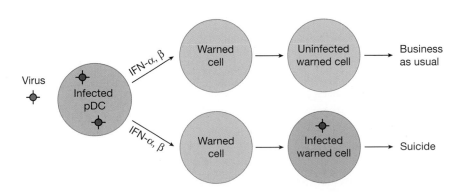

can exist in several stages of readiness. Resting NK cells produce some cytokines and can kill, but they produce larger quantities of cytokines and can kill better if they are activated. **Several signals have been identified that can activate natural killer cells, and each of these signals is generated only when the body is under attack.** During a viral attack, NK cells can be activated by IFN-α and IFN-β, given off by other immune system cells. And when bacteria invade, NK cells can be activated when their surface receptors detect the bacterial cell membrane component LPS.

Natural killer cells can destroy some tumor cells, virus-infected cells, bacteria, parasites, and fungi. They kill these cells by forcing them to commit suicide. In some cases, NK cells employ an "injection system" that uses **perforin** proteins to deliver "suicide" enzymes (e.g., **granzyme B**) into a target cell. In other situations, a protein called **Fas ligand** on the NK cell surface interacts with a protein called Fas on the surface of its target, signaling the target cell to self-destruct.

The method NK cells employ to identify their targets is quite different from that of killer T cells. **Natural killer cells do not have T cell receptors – the receptors that are constructed by mixing and matching gene segments.** The surface receptors that natural killer cells use for target recognition are of two types: **activating receptors** which, when engaged, motivate the NK cell to kill, and **inhibitory receptors** which, when engaged, encourage it not to kill.

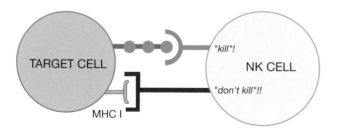

The "don't kill" signal is conveyed by inhibitory receptors that recognize class I MHC molecules on the surface of a potential target cell. Class I MHC molecules are found in varying amounts on the surface of most healthy cells in our bodies. Consequently, the presence of this surface molecule is an indication that a cell is doing okay. In contrast, **the "kill" signals involve interactions between the activating receptors on the surface of an NK cell and unusual carbohydrates or proteins on the surface of a target cell.** These peculiar surface molecules act as flags which indicate that the target cell has been "stressed," usually because it has been infected by a virus

or is becoming cancerous. **It is the balance between the "kill" and the "don't kill" signals which determines whether an NK cell will destroy its target.**

Now, why do you think it would be a good idea to have NK cells destroy cells that do <u>not</u> express class I MHC molecules? You remember that by examining peptides displayed by class I MHC proteins, killer T cells are able to "look inside" cells to see if anything is wrong. But what if some clever virus were to turn off expression of MHC molecules in the cells it infects? Wouldn't those virus-infected cells then be "invisible" to killer T cells? Indeed they would be. So, in those cases, it would be great to have another weapon that could kill virus-infected cells which don't display MHC molecules on their surface. And that's just what natural killer cells can do.

THE INNATE IMMUNE SYSTEM – A COOPERATIVE EFFORT

To make the innate system work efficiently, there must be cooperation between players. For example, neutrophils are on call from the blood. And who does the calling? The sentinel cell, the macrophage. So here we have a defense strategy in which "garbage collectors" alert the "hired guns" when their help is needed. Indeed, cooperation between macrophages and neutrophils is essential for mounting an effective defense against invading microbes. Without macrophages to summon them to sites of attack, neutrophils would just go around and around in the blood. And without neutrophils, macrophages would be hard pressed to deal with sizable infections.

Also, during a bacterial infection, molecules like LPS bind to receptors on the surface of natural killer cells, signaling that an attack is on. NK cells then respond by producing significant amounts of IFN-γ.

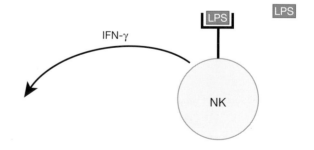

The IFN-γ produced by NK cells can prime macrophages, which can then be hyperactivated when their receptors also bind to LPS.

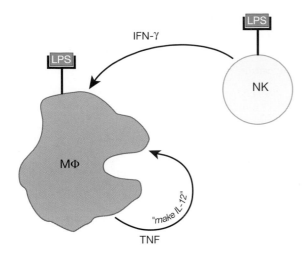

When a macrophage is hyperactivated, it produces lots of TNF. Importantly, a macrophage has receptors on its surface to which this cytokine can bind, so a macrophage can respond to the TNF it produces. And when TNF binds to these receptors, the macrophage begins to secrete IL-12. Together, TNF and IL-12 influence NK cells to increase the amount of IFN-γ they produce. And when there is more IFN-γ around, more macrophages can be primed.

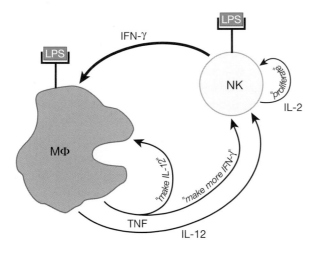

There is something else interesting going on here. **IL-2** is a growth factor that is produced by NK cells. Normally, NK cells don't express the receptor for IL-2, so they don't proliferate in response to this cytokine – even though they are making it. During an infection, however, the TNF produced by macrophages upregulates the expression of IL-2 receptors on the surface of NK cells. Consequently, NK cells can now react to the IL-2 they make and begin to proliferate. As a result of this proliferation, there will soon be many more NK cells to defend against an invasion – and to help activate more macrophages. So

macrophages and NK cells cooperate in several different ways to strengthen the response of the innate system to an attack.

Professional phagocytes and the complement system also work together. As we discussed, complement protein fragments such as iC3b can tag invaders for phagocyte ingestion. But complement opsonization also can play a role in activating macrophages. When C3 fragments that are decorating an invader bind to receptors on the surface of a macrophage, this provides an activation signal for the macrophage which is similar to that supplied by LPS. This is a good idea, because there are invaders that can be opsonized by complement, but which do not make LPS.

Cooperation between the complement system and the phagocytes is not a one-way street. Activated macrophages actually produce several of the most important complement proteins: C3, factor B, and factor D. So in the heat of battle, when complement proteins may be depleted out in the tissues, macrophages can help resupply the complement system. In addition, during an infection, macrophages secrete chemicals that increase the permeability of nearby blood vessels. And when these vessels become leaky, more complement proteins are released into the tissues.

These interactions between phagocytes, NK cells, and the complement proteins are examples of the many ways in which innate system players work together. Only by cooperating with each other can the players on the innate system team respond quickly and strongly to an invasion.

A PROPORTIONAL RESPONSE

In reacting to an attack, our military tries to mount a response which is proportional to the threat. Such a proportional response insures that, on the one hand, resources will not be wasted by overreacting – and, on the other hand, that the reaction will be strong enough to get the job done. The immune system is also set up to provide a proportional response to microbial invasions. For example, the number of macrophages engaged in battle depends on the size of the attack – and the amount of chemicals given off by macrophages to summon neutrophils or activate NK cells depends on how many macrophages are fighting. Consequently, the more serious the invasion, the more macrophages will be involved, and the more neutrophils and NK cells will be mobilized.

Likewise, the larger a bacterial invasion is, the more "danger molecules" such as LPS will be present at the battle scene. And the more LPS there is, the more NK cells will be activated to produce battle cytokines such as IFN-γ, which help activate macrophages. Because the magnitude of the immune response is directly linked to the seriousness of the attack, "the punishment usually fits the crime."

REVIEW

The complement system of proteins functions to destroy invaders and to alert other immune system warriors. For example, complement proteins participate in the construction of membrane attack complexes that can puncture and destroy invading pathogens. Complement proteins also can tag invaders for ingestion by professional phagocytes, and can act as chemoattractants to recruit phagocytic cells to the battle site.

Complement proteins are present in high concentrations in the blood and in the tissues, so they are always ready to go. This is one of the most important features of the complement system: It works really fast. However, for the complement system to spring into action, it must first be activated. Activation by the alternative (spontaneous) pathway simply requires that a complement protein fragment, C3b, bind to an amino or hydroxyl group on an invader. Because these chemical groups are ubiquitous, the default option in this system is death: Any surface that is not protected against binding by complement fragments will be targeted for destruction. Fortunately, there are multiple mechanisms which protect human cells from complement attack.

In addition to the alternative activation pathway, which can be visualized as grenades going off randomly here and there, there is a second pathway for activating the complement system that is more directed: the lectin activation pathway. In this system, a protein called mannose-binding lectin attaches to mannose, a carbohydrate molecule found on the surface of common pathogens. Then, a protein that is bound to the mannose-binding lectin sets off the complement chain reaction on the surface of the invader. Consequently, the mannose-binding lectin acts as a "guidance system" which targets the complement "bombs" to invaders that have distinctive carbohydrate molecules on their surfaces.

Macrophages and neutrophils are professional phagocytes. In tissues, macrophages have a relatively long lifetime. This makes sense because macrophages act as sentinels that patrol the periphery. Most of the time, macrophages just eat dead cells and debris. However, if they find an invader, they become activated. In this activated state, they can present antigens to T cells, they can send out signals that recruit other immune system cells to help in the struggle, and they can become vicious killers.

In contrast to sentinel macrophages, which reside beneath the surface of all the parts of our body that are exposed to the outside world, most neutrophils can be found in the blood – where they are on call in case of attack. Whereas macrophages are quite versatile, neutrophils mainly do one thing – kill. Neutrophils use cellular adhesion molecules to exit blood vessels at sites of inflammation, and as they exit, they are activated to become killers. Fortunately, these cells only live about five days. This limits the damage they can do to healthy tissues once an invader has been vanquished. On the other hand, if the attack is prolonged, there are plenty more neutrophils that can exit the blood and help out.

The innate system is programmed to react to danger signals that are characteristic of commonly encountered pathogens or pathogen-infected cells. Immune system cells are equipped with pattern-recognition receptors that detect common signatures of whole classes of bacteria and viruses. These PRRs also recognize signals given off by dying cells. When these danger signals are detected, sentinel cells such as macrophages respond by producing battle cytokines that alert other cells and prepare them to repulse the attack.

In response to a viral infection, the pattern-recognition receptors of most cells in the body can trigger the production of type I interferons, IFN-α or IFN-β. These proteins function as warning proteins. When they bind to IFN receptors on nearby cells, they prepare these cells to be on their guard against attack by viruses. In preparation, the warned cells produce proteins that will limit the ability of the virus to replicate inside them. And if they are attacked, they are prepared to commit suicide. As a result of this altruistic act, the infected cells and the viruses within them both are destroyed. One of the body's sentinel cells, the plasmacytoid dendritic cell, can produce huge quantities of type I interferons when infected by a virus. For this reason, pDCs are important players in the innate immune system's defense against a viral attack.

The natural killer cell is another player on the innate team which is on call from the blood. These cells are a cross between a killer T cell and a helper T cell. NK cells resemble helper T cells in that they secrete cytokines which affect the function of both the innate and adaptive immune systems. And like cytotoxic lymphocytes, natural killer cells can destroy infected cells. However, in contrast to CTLs, which select their targets by surveying peptides displayed by class I MHC molecules, NK cells focus on killing cells that do not express class I MHC molecules – especially stressed cells that have lost class I MHC expression due to a viral infection.

Phagocytes and the complement proteins provide an immediate response to an attack because these weapons are already in place. As the battle continues, signals given off by the innate system recruit even more defenders from the blood stream, and the innate system warriors cooperate to strengthen the defense. By working together, members of the innate system team provide a fast and effective response to common invaders. Importantly, the system is designed to elicit a defense which avoids overreaction, yet is adequate to the task.

SUMMARY FIGURE

In this figure, I have summarized some of the concepts we discussed in this lecture. For clarity, I have chosen a macrophage as a representative of the professional phagocytes, a bacterium as an example of an invader which can reproduce without entering human cells, and a virus as an example of an invader which must enter a human cell to complete its life cycle. After Lectures 3, 4, and 6, I will expand this figure to include players from the adaptive immune system as they take the field.

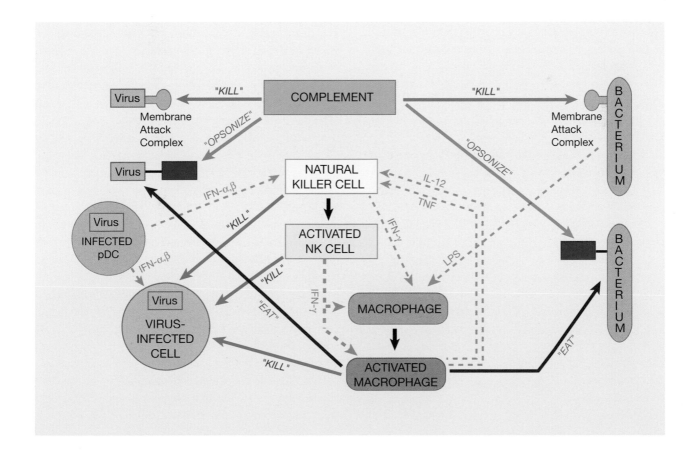

THOUGHT QUESTIONS

1. What is the fundamental difference between the way the complement system is activated by the alternative pathway and the way it is activated by the lectin activation pathway?

2. How do macrophages and natural killer cells tell friend from foe (i.e., how do they select their targets)?

3. Imagine a splinter has punctured your big toe, and that Gram-negative bacteria which produce LPS have invaded the tissues surrounding the splinter. Sketch the likely sequence of events in which the various players of the innate system team deal with this bacterial invasion.

4. Discuss the ways the innate system can protect against a virus attack.

5. Give examples of the cooperation between players on the innate system team, and tell why this cooperation is important.

LECTURE 3 — B Cells and Antibodies

HEADS UP!

B cells and the antibodies they produce are part of the adaptive immune system. B cells must be activated before they can make antibodies. "Fail-safe" mechanisms help prevent inappropriate B cell activation, and the principle of clonal selection insures that only those B cells which make antibodies appropriate to defend against an invader are mobilized. A "mix-and-match" scheme is used to construct the genes that encode a B cell's antibodies, and during the course of an attack, B cells can upgrade the antibodies they produce to mount a more targeted defense.

INTRODUCTION

Microbes such as bacteria and viruses are always mutating. Just as mutations in bacteria can render them resistant to certain antibiotics, mutations also can change microbes in ways that make them better able to resist immune defenses. When this happens, the immune system must "adapt" by producing new counter-weapons in order to keep the mutated microbe from taking over. Indeed, a chess match has been going on for millions of years in which the immune systems of animals constantly have been "upgraded" in response to novel weapons fielded by microbial attackers. The most striking upgrade of the immune system began about 200 million years ago, when, in fish, evolution led to the precursor of what might be called the "ultimate defense" – a system so adaptable that, in principle, it can protect against any possible invader. This defense, the adaptive immune system, has reached its most sophisticated form in humans. Indeed, without

an immune system which can recognize and adapt to deal with unusual invaders, human life would not be possible.

In this lecture, we will focus on one of the most important components of the adaptive immune system: the B cell. Like all the other blood cells, B cells are born in the bone marrow, where they descend from stem cells. About one billion B cells are produced each day during the entire life of a human, so even old guys like me have lots of freshly made B cells. During their early days in the marrow, B cells select gene segments coding for the two proteins that make up their B cell receptors (BCRs), and these receptors then take up their positions on the surface of the B cell. The antibody molecule is almost identical to the B cell receptor, except that it lacks the protein sequences at the tip of the heavy chain which anchor the BCR to the outside of the cell. Lacking this anchor, the antibody molecule is exported out of the B cell, and is free to travel around the body to do its thing.

THE B CELL RECEPTOR

I want to tell you a little about the process of selecting gene segments to make a B cell receptor. I think you'll find it interesting – especially if you like to gamble. **The BCR is made up of two kinds of proteins, the heavy chain (Hc) and the light chain (Lc), and each of these proteins is encoded by genes that are assembled from gene segments.** The gene segments that will be chosen to make up the final Hc gene are located on chromosome 14, and each B cell has two chromosome 14s (one from Mom and one from Dad). This raises a bit of a problem, because, as we discussed earlier, each B cell makes only one kind of antibody. Therefore, because there are two sets of Hc segments, it is necessary to "silence" the segments on one chromosome 14 to keep a B cell from making two different Hc proteins. Of course, Mother Nature could have chosen to make one chromosome a "dummy," so that the other would always be the one that was used – but she didn't. That would have been too boring. Instead, she came up with a much sweeter scheme, which I picture as a game of cards with the two chromosomes as players. It's a game of "winner takes all" in which each player tries to rearrange its cards (gene segments) until it finds an arrangement that works. The first player to do this wins.

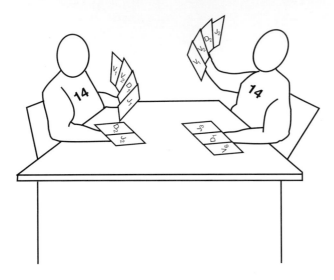

You remember from the first lecture that the finished heavy chain protein is assembled by pasting together four separate gene segments (V, D, J, and C), and that lined up along chromosome 14 are multiple, slightly different copies of each kind of segment.

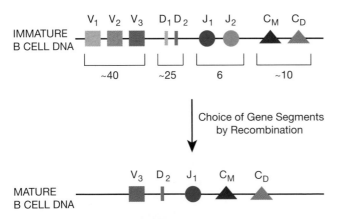

The players in this card game first choose one each of the possible D and J segments, and these are joined together by deleting the DNA sequences in between them. Then one of the many V segments is chosen, and this "card" is joined to the DJ segment, again by deleting the DNA in between. Right next to the J segment is a string of gene segments (C_M, C_D, etc.) that code for various constant regions. By default, the constant regions for IgM and IgD are used to make the BCR, just because they are first in line. Immunologists call these joined-together gene segments a "gene rearrangement," but it is really more about cutting and pasting than rearranging. Anyway, the result is that the chosen V, D, and J segments and the constant region segments all end up adjacent to each other on the chromosome.

Next, the rearranged gene segments are tested. What's the test? Protein translation stops when the ribosome encounters one of the three stop codons. So if the gene segments are not joined up just right (in frame), the protein translation machinery will encounter a stop codon and terminate protein assembly somewhere in the middle of the heavy chain. If this happens, the result is a useless little piece of protein. In fact, you can calculate that each player only has about one chance in nine of assembling a winning combination of gene segments that will produce a full-length Hc protein. Immunologists call such a combination of gene segments a **productive rearrangement**. If one of the chromosomes that is playing this game ends up with a productive rearrangement, that chromosome is used to construct the winning Hc protein. This heavy chain protein is then transported to the cell surface, where it signals to the losing chromosome that the game is over. The details of how the signal is sent, and how it stops the rearrangement of gene segments on the other chromosome remain to be discovered. However, it is thought to have something to do with changing the conformation of the DNA on the losing chromosome – so that it no longer is accessible to the cut-and-paste machinery.

Since each player only has about a one in nine chance of success, you may be wondering what happens if both chromosomes fail to assemble gene segments that result in a productive rearrangement. Well, the B cell dies. That's right, it commits suicide! It's a high-stakes game, because a B cell that cannot express a receptor is totally useless.

If the heavy chain rearrangement is productive, the baby B cell proliferates for a bit, and then the light chain players step up to the table. The rules of their game are similar to those of the heavy chain game, but there is an additional test which must be passed to win: The completed heavy and light chain proteins must fit together properly to make a complete antibody. If the B cell fails to productively rearrange heavy and light chains, or if the Hcs and Lcs don't match up correctly, the B cell commits suicide.

The result of this contest is that although a B cell can display as many as 100 000 BCRs on its surface, **every** mature B cell produces one and only one kind of BCR or antibody, made up of one and only one kind of Hc and Lc. Nevertheless, because a mix and match strategy is used to make the final Hc and Lc genes of each B cell, the receptors on different B cells are so diverse that collectively, our B cells can probably recognize any organic molecule that could exist. When you consider how many molecules that might be, the fact that a simple scheme like this can create such diversity is truly breathtaking.

HOW THE BCR SIGNALS

Immunologists call the antigen that a given B cell's receptors recognize its **cognate antigen**, and the tiny region of the cognate antigen that a BCR actually binds to is called its **epitope**. For example, if a B cell's cognate antigen happens to be a protein on the surface of the flu virus, the epitope will be the part of that protein (usually 6–12 amino acids) to which the BCR actually binds. When the BCR recognizes the epitope for which it is matched, it must signal this recognition to the nucleus of the B cell, where genes involved in activating the B cell can be turned on or off. But how does this BCR "antenna" send a signal to the nucleus that it has found its epitope? At first sight it would appear that this could be a bit of a problem, because, as you can see from this figure, the part of the heavy chain that extends through the cell membrane into the interior of the cell is only a few amino acids in length – way too short to do any serious signaling.

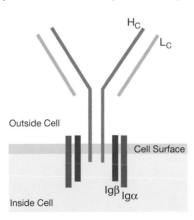

To make it possible for the external part of the BCR to signal what it has seen, B cells are equipped with two accessory proteins, Igα and Igβ, which associate with the heavy chain protein and protrude into the inside of the cell. Thus, **the complete B cell receptor really has two parts: the Hc/Lc part outside the cell that recognizes the** antigen but can't signal, plus the Igα and Igβ proteins that can signal, but which are totally blind to what's going on outside the cell.

To generate an activation signal, many BCRs must be brought close together on the surface of the B cell. When BCRs are clustered like this, immunologists say they are **crosslinked** – although the receptors really are not linked together. B cell receptors can be clustered, for example, when they bind to an epitope that is present multiple times on a single antigen (e.g., a protein in which a sequence of amino acids is repeated many times).

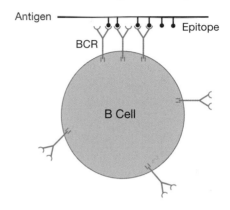

Crosslinking of BCRs also can result when BCRs bind to epitopes on individual antigens that are close together on the surface of an invader. Indeed, the surfaces of most bacteria, viruses, and parasites are composed of many copies of a few different proteins. So if a B cell's receptors recognize an epitope on one of these proteins, lots of BCRs can be clustered. Indeed, the requirement for crosslinking is one way B cells focus on common enemies. Finally, B cell receptors also can be brought together by binding to epitopes on antigens that are clumped together (e.g., a clump of proteins). Regardless of how it is accomplished, **crosslinking of B cell receptors is essential for B cell activation.** Here's why.

The tails of the Igα and Igβ proteins interact with signaling molecules inside the cell. And when enough of these interactions are concentrated in one region, an enzymatic chain reaction is initiated which sends a message to the nucleus of the cell saying, "BCR engaged." So the trick to sending this message is to get lots of Igα and Igβ molecules together – and that's exactly what crosslinking a B cell's receptors does. **The clustering of BCRs brings enough Igα and Igβ molecules together to set off the chain reaction that sends the "BCR engaged" signal.** So BCR crosslinking is key.

You remember from the last lecture that fragments of the complement proteins (e.g., C3b) can bind to (opsonize) invaders. This tag indicates that the invader has been recognized as dangerous by the innate immune system, and invites innate system players such as macrophages to destroy the opsonized invader. It turns out that antigens opsonized by complement fragments also can alert the adaptive immune system. Here's how.

In addition to the B cell receptor and its associated signaling molecules, there is another protein on the surface of a B cell that can play an important role in signaling. This protein is a receptor that can bind to complement fragments which are decorating an invader. Consequently, for an opsonized antigen, there are two receptors on a B cell that can bind to the antigen: the BCR which recognizes a specific epitope on the antigen, and the complement receptor that recognizes the "decorations." When this happens, the opsonized antigen acts as a "clamp" that brings the BCR and the complement receptor together on the surface of the B cell.

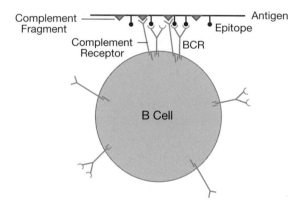

When the BCR and the complement receptor are brought together in this way by opsonized antigen, the signal that the BCR sends is greatly amplified. What this means in practice is that the number of BCRs that must be clustered to send the "receptor engaged" signal to the nucleus is decreased at least 100-fold. **Because the complement receptor can have such a dramatic effect on signaling, it is called a co-receptor.** The function of this co-receptor is especially important during the initial stages of an attack, when the amount of antigen available to crosslink B cell receptors is limited. **Recognition of opsonized invaders by the B cell's co-receptor serves to make B cells exquisitely sensitive to antigens which the innate system already has identified as dangerous. This is an excellent example of the "instructive" function of the innate system. Indeed, the decision on whether an invader is dangerous or not usually is made by the innate, not the adaptive system.**

HOW B CELLS ARE ACTIVATED

To produce antibodies, B cells must first be activated. B cells that have never been activated by encountering their cognate antigen are called **naive** or **virgin B cells**. An example would be a B cell that can recognize the smallpox virus, but which happens to reside in a human who has never been exposed to smallpox. In contrast, B cells that have encountered their cognate antigen and have been activated are called **experienced B cells**. There are two ways that naive B cells can be activated to defend us against invaders. One is completely dependent on the assistance of helper T cells (**T cell-dependent activation**) and the second is more or less independent of T cell help (**T cell-independent activation**).

T-cell dependent activation

Activation of a naive B cell requires two signals. The first is the clustering of the B cell's receptors and their associated signaling molecules. However, just having its receptors crosslinked is not enough to fully activate a B cell – a second signal is required. Immunologists call this the **co-stimulatory signal**. In T cell-dependent activation, this second signal is supplied by a helper T (Th) cell. The best studied co-stimulatory signal involves direct contact between a B cell and a Th cell. On the surface of activated helper T cells are proteins called **CD40L**. If a B cell's receptors have been crosslinked, and if CD40L plugs into (ligates) a protein called **CD40** on the surface of the B cell, that B cell will be activated.

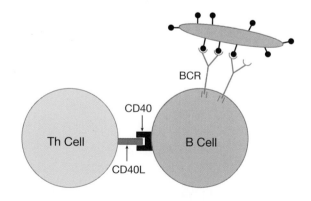

The interaction between these two proteins, CD40 and CD40L, is clearly very important for B cell activation. Humans who have a genetic defect in either of these proteins are unable to mount a T cell-dependent antibody defense.

T cell-independent activation

In response to certain antigens, virgin B cells can also be activated with little or no T cell help. This mode of activation is termed T cell-independent. What these antigens have in common is that they have repeated epitopes which can crosslink a ton of B cell receptors. A good example of such an antigen is a carbohydrate of the type found on the surface of many bacterial cells. A carbohydrate molecule is made up of many repeating units, much like beads on a string. If each "bead" is recognized by the BCR as its epitope, the string of beads can bring together many, many BCRs. The crosslinking of such a large number of BCRs can partially substitute for co-stimulation by CD40L, and can cause a B cell to proliferate. But to be fully activated and produce antibodies, a naive B cell must receive a second signal.

For T cell-independent activation, this second "key" is an unambiguous "danger signal" – a clear indication that an attack is on. For example, in addition to their BCRs, B cells express Toll-like receptors, and these TLRs can alert a B cell to danger and provide the second key needed for activation. What is important here is that if a B cell has BCRs that can recognize a molecule with repeated epitopes like, for example, your own DNA, it may proliferate, but fortunately, no anti-DNA antibodies will be produced. The reason is that your immune system is not engaged in a battle with your own DNA, so there will be no danger signals to provide the necessary co-stimulation. On the other hand, if the innate immune system is battling a bacterial infection, and a B cell's receptors recognize a carbohydrate antigen with repeated epitopes on the surface of the bacterial invader, that B cell will produce antibodies – because danger signals from the battleground can supply the second key needed for complete B cell activation. Of course, as is true of T cell-dependent activation, T cell-independent activation is antigen specific: Only those B cells whose receptors recognize the repeated epitope will be activated.

One advantage of T cell-independent activation is that B cells can jump right into the fray without having to wait for helper T cells to be activated. The result is a speedier antibody response. Most B cells that are activated without T cell help are found in the spleen. These B cells can mount a rapid defense against bacteria like *Streptococcus pneumoniae* by making IgM antibodies that recognize epitopes on the polysaccharide capsule that surrounds the bacterium. The importance of this T cell-independent activation is demonstrated by the fact that humans who have had their spleens removed are at high risk for infection by *Streptococcus pneumoniae* and other encapsulated bacteria.

There is something else important going on here. Helper T cells only recognize protein antigens – the peptides presented by class II MHC molecules. Consequently, if all B cell activation required T cell help, the entire adaptive immune system would be focused on proteins. This wouldn't be so great, because many of the most common invaders have carbohydrates or fats on their surface that are not found on the surface of human cells. Therefore, these carbohydrates and fats make excellent targets for recognition by the immune system. So by allowing some antigens to activate B cells without T cell help, Mother Nature did a wonderful thing: She increased the universe of antigens that the adaptive immune system can react against to include not only proteins, but carbohydrates and fats as well.

The logic of B cell activation

You may be asking yourself: Why does B cell activation require two signals? Wouldn't things go more quickly if all a B cell needed for activation was crosslinking of its receptors? Yes, this probably would speed up antibody production, but it would also be way too dangerous. Because of the diversity of B cell receptors, there is essentially no limit on what they can recognize – including our own proteins, carbohydrates, and fats. Most B cells which can recognize our own molecules are eliminated shortly after they are born in the bone marrow (much more on this in Lecture 9). However, this screening process is not 100% effective, and there are self-reactive B cells in circulation which could cause autoimmune disease if they produced antibodies (autoantibodies). To guard against this possibility there is a fail-safe mechanism in place which allows B cell activation only when there is real danger. That's where the second signal comes in. For T cell-dependent activation, the B cell and the Th cell must agree that there is a threat before the B cell can receive this second signal. For T cell-independent activation, the second signal is a clear indication that there has been an invasion – a dangerous situation which warrants B cell activation.

Polyclonal activation

In addition to T cell-dependent and T cell-independent activation of B cells, there is another, "unnatural" way that B cells can be activated. In this case, the antigen, usually called a **mitogen**, binds to molecules on the B cell surface that are not B cell receptors, and brings these molecules together. When this happens, BCRs that are associated with these molecules also can be clustered. In contrast to T cell-dependent and T cell-independent activation, this **polyclonal activation** does not depend on the cognate antigen recognized by the BCR – the BCR just comes along for the ride. In this way, many different B cells with many different specificities can be activated by a single mitogen. Indeed, mitogens are favorite tools of immunologists, because they can be used to activate a lot of B cells simultaneously, making it easier to study events that take place during activation.

One example of a mitogen is the highly repetitive structure that makes up the surface of certain parasites. During a parasitic infection, the molecules that make up these structures can bind to receptors (mitogen receptors) on the surface of B cells and cluster them. And when the mitogen receptors are clustered in this way, the cell's BCRs also are dragged together. The result is polyclonal activation of B cells. But why would the immune system want to react to a parasitic attack by activating B cells whose BCRs do not even recognize the parasite? The answer is that this is <u>not</u> something the immune system was designed to do! By activating a bunch of B cells that will produce irrelevant antibodies, the parasite seeks to distract the immune system from focusing on the job at hand – destroying the parasitic invader. So **polyclonal activation of B cells by a mitogen actually is an example of the immune system gone wrong – a subject we will discuss at length in another lecture.**

CLASS SWITCHING

Once B cells have been activated, and have proliferated to build up their numbers, they are ready for the next stage in their life: maturation. Maturation can be divided roughly into three steps: **class switching**, in which a B cell can change the class of antibody it produces; **somatic hypermutation**, in which the rearranged genes for the B cell receptor can mutate to increase the average affinity of the BCRs for their cognate antigen; and a "career decision," during which the B cell decides whether to become an antibody factory (a **plasma B cell**) or a **memory B cell**. The exact order of these maturation steps varies, and some B cells may skip one or more steps altogether.

When a virgin B cell is first activated, it produces mainly IgM antibodies – the default antibody class. B cells also can produce IgD antibodies. However, IgD antibodies represent only a tiny fraction of the circulating antibodies in a human, and it is unclear whether they actually perform any significant function in the immune defense. You remember that an antibody's class is determined by the constant (Fc) region of its heavy chain – the "tail" of the antibody molecule, if you will. Interestingly, the same heavy chain messenger RNA is used to make both IgM and IgD, but the mRNA is spliced one way to yield an M-type constant region and another way to produce a D-type constant region.

As a B cell matures, it has the opportunity to change the class of antibody it makes to one of the other antibody classes: IgG, IgE, or IgA. Located just next to the gene segment on chromosome 14 that encodes the constant region for IgM are the constant region segments for IgG, IgE, and IgA. So all that a B cell has to do to switch its class is to cut off the IgM constant region DNA and paste on one of the other constant regions (deleting the DNA in between). Special switching signals that allow this cutting and pasting to take place are located between the constant region segments. For example, here's what happens when a B cell switches from an IgM constant region (C_M in this drawing) to an IgG constant region (C_G):

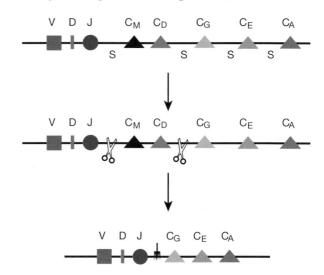

The net result of class switching is that although the part of the antibody that binds to the antigen (the Fab region) remains the same, the antibody gets a new Fc region. This is an important change, because it is the constant region which determines how the antibody will function.

ANTIBODY CLASSES AND THEIR FUNCTIONS

Let's take a look at the four main classes of antibodies: IgM, IgA, IgG, and IgE. As you will see, because of the unique structure of its constant region, each antibody class is particularly well suited to perform certain duties.

IgM antibodies

IgM antibodies were the first class of antibodies to evolve, and even "lower" vertebrates (my apologies to the animal rights folks) have adaptive immune systems that produce IgM antibodies. So it makes sense that in humans, **when naive B cells are first activated, they mainly make IgM antibodies.** You may remember that an IgG antibody looks roughly like this.

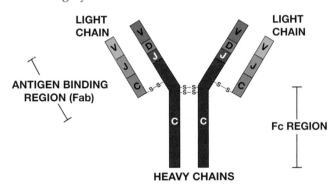

In contrast, an IgM antibody is like five IgG antibody molecules all stuck together. It's really m̲assive!

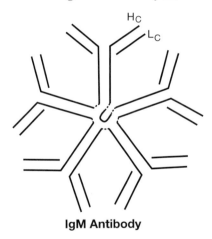

IgM Antibody

Producing IgM antibodies early during an infection actually is quite smart, because IgM antibodies are very good at activating the complement cascade (immunologists call this **fixing complement**). Here's how it works.

In the blood and tissues, some of the complement proteins (about 30 of them!) get together to form a big complex called C1. Despite its size, this complex of proteins cannot activate the complement cascade because it's bound to an inhibitor molecule. However, if two or more C1 complexes are brought close together, their inhibitors fall off, and the C1 molecules can then initiate a cascade of chemical reactions that produces a C3 convertase. Once this happens, the complement system is in business because a C3 convertase converts C3 to C3b, setting up

an amplification loop that produces more and more C3b. So the trick to activating the complement system by this **classical (antibody-dependent) pathway** is to bring two or more of the C1 complexes together – and that's just what an IgM antibody can do.

Once the antigen-binding regions of an IgM antibody have bound to an invader, C1 complexes can bind to the Fc regions of the antibody. Because each IgM antibody has five Fc regions close together (this is the important point), two C1 complexes can bind to the Fc regions of the same IgM antibody, bringing the complexes close enough together to set off the complement cascade. So the sequence of events is: **The IgM antibody binds to the invader, several C1 molecules bind to the Fc region of the IgM antibody, their inhibitors are released, and the C1 molecules trigger the complement chain reaction on the invader's surface.**

The reason the classical activation pathway is so useful is that some clever bacteria have evolved coats which resist the attachment of complement proteins. However, B cells can produce antibodies which will bind to essentially any coat a bacterium might put on. Consequently, antibodies can extend the range of the complement system by helping attach complement proteins to the surface of wily bacteria. This is a nice example of the innate immune system (the complement proteins) cooperating with the adaptive immune system (IgM antibodies) to help destroy an invader. In fact, the term "complement" was coined by immunologists when they first discovered that antibodies were much more effective in dealing with invaders if they were "complemented" by other proteins – the complement proteins.

The alternative (spontaneous) complement activation pathway that we talked about in the last lecture is totally non-specific: Any unprotected surface is fair game. In contrast, the classical (antibody-dependent) activation pathway is quite specific: Only those antigens to which the antibody binds will be targeted for complement attack. In this system, the antibody identifies the invader, and the complement proteins do the dirty work.

Certain "subclasses" of IgG antibodies also can fix complement, because C1 can bind to the Fc region of these antibodies. However, IgG antibodies are real wimps, with only one Fc region per molecule. So bringing two C1 complexes close enough together to get things started requires that two molecules of IgG bind very close together on the surface of the invading pathogen – and this is likely to happen only when there is a lot of IgG around. So, **early in** an infection, when antibodies are just beginning to be made, IgM antibodies have a great advantage over IgG antibodies because they fix complement so efficiently. In addition, IgM antibodies are very good at neutralizing viruses by binding to them and preventing them from infecting cells. Because of these properties, IgM is the perfect "first antibody" to defend against viral or bacterial infections.

IgG antibodies

IgG antibodies come in a number of different subclasses that have slightly different Fc regions and therefore, different functions. For example, one subclass of human IgG antibodies, IgG1, is very good at binding to invaders to opsonize them for ingestion by professional phagocytes. This is because macrophages and neutrophils have receptors on their surfaces that can bind to the Fc portion of IgG1 antibodies once those antibodies have bound to an invader.

Another IgG subclass, IgG3, fixes complement better than any other IgG subclass. In addition, natural killer cells have receptors on their surface that can bind to the Fc region of IgG3 antibodies. As a result, IgG3 can form a bridge between an NK cell and its target by binding to the target cell (e.g., a virus-infected cell) with its Fab region, and to the NK cell with its Fc region. Not only does this bring the NK cell close to its target, but having its Fc receptors bound actually stimulates an NK cell to be a more effective killer. **This process is called antibody-dependent cellular cytotoxicity (ADCC). In ADCC, the NK cell does the killing, but the antibody identifies the target.**

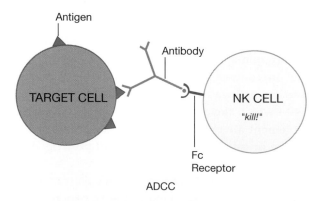

ADCC

Like IgM antibodies, IgG antibodies also are very good at neutralizing viruses. Moreover, IgG antibodies are unique in that they can pass from the mother's blood into the blood of the fetus by way of the placenta. This provides the fetus with a supply of IgG antibodies to tide it over until it begins to produce its own – several months

after birth. This extended protection is possible because IgG antibodies are the longest lived antibody class, with a half-life of about three weeks. In contrast, IgM antibodies have a half-life of only about one day.

The "G" in IgG stands for "gamma," and IgG antibodies are sometimes called **gamma globulins**. If there is a possibility that you have been exposed to an infectious agent, say hepatitis A virus, your doctor may recommend that you get a gamma globulin shot. These shots are prepared by pooling together antibodies from a large number of people, at least some of whom have been infected with hepatitis A virus – and therefore are making antibodies against the virus. The hope is that these "borrowed" antibodies will neutralize most of the virus to which you have been exposed, and that this treatment will help keep the viral infection under control until your own immune system can be activated.

IgA antibodies

Here's a question for you: What is the most abundant antibody class in the human body? No, it's not IgG. It's IgA. This is really a trick question, because I told you earlier that IgG was the most abundant antibody class in the blood – which is true. It turns out, however, that we humans synthesize more IgA antibodies than all the other antibody classes combined. Why so much IgA? Because **IgA is the main antibody class that guards the mucosal surfaces of the body**, and a human has about 400 square meters of mucosal surfaces to defend. These include the digestive, respiratory, and reproductive tracts. So although there aren't a lot of IgA antibodies circulating in the blood, there are tons of them protecting the mucosal surfaces. Indeed, about 80% of the B cells that are located beneath these surfaces produce IgA antibodies.

One reason IgA antibodies are so good at defending against invaders that would like to penetrate the mucosal barrier is that each IgA molecule is rather like two IgG molecules held together by a "clip."

"Clip" L_C H_C

IgA Antibody

The clipped-together tail structure of IgA antibodies is responsible for several important properties of this antibody class. **This clip functions as a "passport" that facilitates the transport of IgA antibodies across the** intestinal wall and out into the intestine. Moreover, this unique structure makes IgA antibodies resistant to acids and enzymes found in the digestive tract. Once inside the intestine, IgA antibodies can "coat" invading pathogens and keep them from attaching to the intestinal cells they would like to infect. In addition, whereas each IgG molecule has two antigen-binding regions, the "dimeric" IgA molecule has four Fab regions to bind antigens. **Consequently, dimeric IgA antibodies are very good at collecting pathogens together into clumps that are large enough to be swept out of the body with mucus or feces.** In fact, rejected bacteria make up about 30% of normal fecal matter.

All together, these qualities make IgA antibodies perfect for guarding mucosal surfaces. Indeed, **it is the IgA class of antibodies that is secreted into the milk of nursing mothers. These IgA antibodies coat the baby's intestinal mucosa and provide protection against pathogens that the baby ingests.** This makes sense, because many of the microbes that babies encounter are taken in through their mouths – babies like to put their mouths on everything, you know.

Although IgA antibodies are very effective against mucosal invaders, they are totally useless at fixing complement: C1 won't even bind to an IgA antibody's Fc region. Again we see that **the constant region of an antibody determines both its class and its function.** This lack of complement-fixing activity is actually a good thing. If IgA antibodies could initiate the complement reaction, our mucosal surfaces would be in a constant state of inflammation in response to both pathogenic and non-pathogenic microbes. And, of course, having chronically inflamed intestines would not be all that great. So IgA antibodies mainly function as "passive" antibodies that block the attachment of invaders to cells that line our mucosal surfaces and usher these unwanted guests out of the body.

IgE antibodies

The IgE antibody class has an interesting history. In the early 1900s, a French physician named Charles Richet was sailing with Prince Albert of Monaco (Grace Kelly's father-in-law). The prince remarked to Richet that it was very strange how some people react violently to the toxin in the sting of the Portuguese man-of-war, and that this phenomenon might be worthy of study.

Richet took his advice, and when he returned to Paris, he decided, as a first experiment, to test how much toxin was required to kill a dog. Don't ask me why he decided to use dogs in his experiments. Maybe there were a lot of stray dogs around back then, or perhaps he just didn't like working with mice. Anyway, the experiment was a success and he was able to determine the amount of toxin that was lethal. However, many of the dogs he used in this first experiment survived, because they didn't receive the lethal dose. Not being one who would waste a good dog, Richet decided to inject these "leftovers" with the toxin again to see what would happen. His expectation was that these animals might have become immune to the effects of the toxin, and that the first injection would have provided protection (prophylaxis) against a second injection. You can imagine his surprise then, when all the dogs died – even the ones that received tiny amounts of toxin in the second injection. Since the first injection had the opposite effect of protection, Richet coined the word **anaphylaxis** to describe this phenomenon ("ana" is a prefix meaning "opposite"). Richet continued these studies on anaphylactic shock, and in 1913, he received the Nobel Prize for his work. I guess one lesson from this is that if a prince suggests you should study something, you might want to take his advice seriously!

Immunologists now know that **anaphylactic shock is caused by mast cells degranulating.** Like macrophages, mast cells are white blood cells that are stationed beneath all exposed surfaces (e.g., beneath the skin or the mucosal barrier). As blood cells go, mast cells are very long-lived: They can survive for years in our tissues. There they lie in wait to protect us against infection by parasites that have penetrated our barrier defenses.

Stored safely inside mast cells are "granules" that contain all kinds of pre-activated, pharmacologically active chemicals, the most famous of which is histamine. Indeed, a mast cell is so full of these granules that its name is derived from the German word *mastung*, which means "well fed." When a mast cell encounters a parasite, it exports its granules (i.e., it "degranulates"), and dumps the contents of these granules onto the parasite to kill it. Unfortunately, in addition to killing parasites, mast cell degranulation also can cause an allergic reaction, and in extreme cases, anaphylactic shock. Here's how this works.

An antigen (e.g., the man-of-war toxin) that can cause an allergic reaction is called an **allergen**. On the first exposure to an allergen, some people, for reasons that are far from clear, make a lot of IgE antibodies directed against the allergen. Mast cells have receptors (IgE receptors) on their surface that can bind to the Fc region of these IgE antibodies. And when this happens, the mast cells are like bombs waiting to explode.

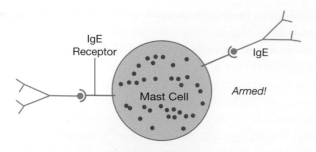

AFTER FIRST EXPOSURE

On a second exposure to the allergen, IgE antibodies that are already bound to the surfaces of mast cells can bind to the allergen. Because allergens usually are proteins with a repeating sequence, they can crosslink many IgE molecules on the mast cell surface, dragging the Fc receptors together. This clustering of Fc receptors is similar to the crosslinking of B cell receptors in that bringing many of these receptors together results in a signal being sent. In this case, however, the signal says "degranulate," and the mast cell responds by dumping its granules into the surrounding tissues.

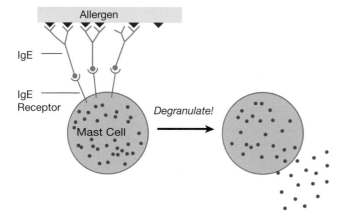

Histamines and other chemicals released from mast cell granules increase capillary permeability so that fluid escapes from the capillaries into the tissue. That's why you get a runny nose and watery eyes when you have an allergic reaction. This is usually a rather local effect, but if the toxin spreads throughout the body and triggers massive degranulation of mast cells, things can get serious. In such a case, the release of fluid from the blood into the tissues can reduce the blood volume so much that the heart no longer can pump efficiently, resulting in a heart attack. In addition, histamine from the granules can cause smooth muscles around the windpipe to contract, making it difficult to breathe. In extreme cases, this contraction can be strong enough to cause suffocation. Most of us don't

have to worry about being stung by a Portuguese man-of-war, but we may need to be wary of bees. Some people make lots of IgE antibodies in response to bee toxin, and for those folks a bee sting can be fatal. Indeed, about 1500 Americans die each year from anaphylactic shock.

This brings us to an interesting question: Why are B cells allowed to switch the class of antibody they make anyway? Wouldn't it be safer just to stick with good old IgM antibodies? I don't think so. Let's suppose you have a viral infection of your respiratory tract, resulting in the common cold. Would you want to be stuck making only IgM antibodies? Certainly not. You'd want a lot of IgA antibodies to be secreted into the mucus that lines your respiratory tract to bind up that virus, and help remove it from your body. On the other hand, if you have a parasitic infection (worms, for example), you'd want IgE antibodies to be produced, because IgE antibodies can cause cells like mast cells to degranulate, making life miserable for those worms. So **the beauty of this system is that the different classes of antibodies are uniquely suited to defend against different invaders.**

ANTIBODY CLASS	ANTIBODY PROPERTIES
IgM	Great complement fixer Good opsonizer First antibody made
IgA	Resistant to stomach acid Protects mucosal surfaces Secreted in milk
IgG	OK complement fixer Good opsonizer Helps NK cell kill (ADCC) Can cross placenta
IgE	Defends against parasites Causes anaphylactic shock Causes allergies

Now suppose Mother Nature could arrange to have your immune system make IgG antibodies when your big toe is infected, IgA antibodies when you have a cold, or IgE antibodies when you have a parasitic infection. Wouldn't that be elegant? Well, it turns out that this is exactly what happens! Here's how it works.

Antibody class switching is controlled by the cytokines that B cells encounter when switching takes place: Certain cytokines or combinations of cytokines influence B cells to switch to one class or another. For example, if B cells class switch in an environment that is rich in IL-4 and IL-5, they preferentially switch their class from IgM to IgE – just right for those worms. On the other hand, if there is a lot of IFN-γ around, B cells switch to produce IgG3 antibodies that are very effective against bacteria and viruses. Or, if a cytokine called TGFβ is present during the class switch, B cells preferentially change from IgM to IgA antibody production – perfect for the common cold. So, to insure that the antibody response will be appropriate for a given invader, all Mother Nature has to do is to arrange to have the right cytokines present when B cells switch classes. But how could she accomplish this?

You remember that helper T cells are "quarterback" cells which direct the immune response. One way they do this is by producing cytokines which influence B cells to make the antibody class that is right to defend against a given invader. To learn how Th cells know which cytokines to make, you'll have to wait for the next three lectures when we discuss antigen presentation and T cell activation and function. But for now, I'll just give you the bottom line: In response to cytokines made by Th cells, B cells can switch from making IgM antibodies to producing one of the other antibody classes. As a result, the adaptive immune system can respond with antibodies tailor-made for each kind of invader – be it a bacterium, a flu virus, or a worm. What could be better than that?!

SOMATIC HYPERMUTATION

As if class switching weren't great enough, there is yet another amazing thing that can happen to B cells as they mature. Normally, the overall mutation rate of DNA in human cells is extremely low – only about one mutated base per 100 million bases per DNA replication cycle. It has to be this low or we'd all end up looking like Star Wars characters with three eyes and six ears. However, in very restricted regions of the chromosomes of B cells – those regions that contain the V, D, and J gene segments – an extremely high rate of mutation can take place. In fact, mutation rates as high as one mutated base per 1000 bases per generation have been measured. We're talking serious mutations here! This high rate of mutation is called **somatic hypermutation**, and it occurs after the V, D, and

J segments have been selected – and usually after class switching has taken place. So somatic hypermutation is a relatively late event in the maturation of B cells. Indeed, B cells that still make IgM antibodies usually have not undergone somatic hypermutation.

What somatic hypermutation does is to change (mutate) the part of the rearranged antibody gene that encodes the antigen-binding region of the antibody. Depending on the mutation there are three possible outcomes: The affinity of the antibody molecule for its cognate antigen may remain unchanged, it may be increased, or it may be decreased. Now comes the neat part. In order for maturing B cells to proliferate, they must continually be re-stimulated by helper T cells. Those B cells whose BCRs have mutated to higher affinity compete more successfully for T cell help. Consequently, they proliferate more frequently than do B cells with lower affinity receptors. Therefore, the result of somatic hypermutation is that you end up with many more B cells whose BCRs bind tightly to their cognate antigen.

By using somatic hypermutation to make changes in the antigen-binding region of a BCR, and by using binding and proliferation to select those mutations that have increased the BCR's affinity for antigen, B cell receptors can be "fine-tuned." The result is a collection of B cells whose receptors have a higher average affinity for their cognate antigen. This whole process is called **affinity maturation**.

So B cells can change their constant (Fc) region by class switching, and their antigen-binding (Fab) region by somatic hypermutation – and these two modifications produce B cells that are better adapted to deal with invaders. The assistance of helper T cells usually is required for B cells to make either of these upgrades. As a result, B cells that are activated without T cell help (e.g., in response to carbohydrates on the surface of a bacterium) generally don't undergo either class switching or somatic hypermutation.

B CELLS MAKE A CAREER CHOICE

The final step in the maturation of a B cell is the choice of profession. This can't be too tough, because a B cell really only has two fates to choose between: to become a **plasma B cell** or a **memory B cell**. **Plasma B cells are antibody factories.** If a B cell decides to become a plasma cell, it usually travels to the spleen or back to the bone marrow, and begins to produce the secreted form of the BCR – the antibody molecule. Some plasma B cells can synthesize 2000 of these antibodies each second. However, as a result of this heroic effort, these plasma B cells only live for a few days. The fact that one plasma B cell can make so many antibody molecules helps the immune system keep up with invaders like bacteria and viruses which multiply very quickly.

Although the B cell's other possible career choice – to become a memory B cell – may not be quite so dramatic as the decision to become a plasma cell, it is extremely important. It is the memory B cell that recalls your first exposure to a pathogen, and helps defend you against subsequent exposures. Immunologists haven't figured out how a B cell "chooses" to become either a memory cell or a plasma cell. However, they do know that the interaction between the co-stimulatory molecule CD40L on the surface of a helper T cell and CD40 on the B cell surface is important in memory cell generation. Indeed, **memory B cells are not produced when B cells are activated without T cell help.**

REVIEW

A B cell's receptors function as the "eyes" of the cell, and actually have two parts: a recognition part (made up of the heavy and light chain proteins), and a signaling part (made up of two other proteins, Igα and Igβ). The final genes that encode the recognition part are made by mixing and matching gene segments. The result is a collection of B cells with receptors so diverse that they probably can recognize any organic molecule in the universe. For these receptors to signal what they have seen requires that multiple BCRs be clustered (crosslinked). This crosslinking brings the Igα and Igβ signaling molecules that are associated with the heavy chains close together. And when enough Igα and Igβ molecules are clustered in this way, a threshold amount of enzymatic activity is reached, and the "receptor engaged" signal is sent to the nucleus of the B cell.

B cells also have co-receptor molecules on their surface which can recognize opsonized antigen. When both the B cell's receptors and the co-receptors are engaged by an antigen, the number of BCRs which must be crosslinked to signal activation is dramatically reduced. Consequently, these co-receptors focus the attention of B cells on antigens that have already been recognized by the innate system as dangerous and which have been opsonized.

Activation of a virgin B cell requires two "keys." Crosslinking of the B cell's receptors is the first key, but a second, "co-stimulatory" key also is required. This key usually is provided by a helper T cell, and involves cell–cell contact, during which CD40L molecules on the surface of a helper T cell bind to CD40 proteins on the surface of a B cell. B cells can also be activated without T cell help. The first requirement for this T cell-independent activation is that a large number of the B cell's receptors must be crosslinked. This typically happens when the surface of an invader is made up of many copies of the antigen to which a B cell's receptors bind (its "cognate" antigen). Although the crosslinking of many B cell receptors is a requisite for T cell-independent activation of a naive B cell, it is not enough. A second, co-stimulatory signal also is needed. This co-stimulation is in the form of a "danger signal" which confirms that an authentic threat exists. By demanding that two keys must be supplied before a B cell can be activated, a fail-safe system is established that guards against inappropriate B cell activation.

IgM antibodies are the first antibodies produced by B cells in response to a pathogen that has not been encountered before. However, as a B cell matures, it can choose to produce a different class of antibody: either IgG, IgA, or IgE. This class switching does not change the antigen-binding (Fab) region of the antibody. Consequently, the antibody recognizes the same antigen before and after its class has been switched.

What does change during class switching is the Fc region of the heavy chain. This is the part of the molecule that determines how the antibody functions, with some functions being better suited to certain invaders than to others. For example, most antibodies can opsonize antigens for phagocyte ingestion – because phagocytes have receptors on their surface that can bind to the Fc region of antibodies which have bound their cognate antigen. Certain classes of antibodies can activate the complement cascade when they bind to antigen, because of the structure of their Fc region. And some antibody classes can facilitate antibody-dependent cellular toxicity by forming a bridge between natural killer cells and invading microbes. Importantly, the choice of antibody class is determined by the cytokines present in the local environment of the B cell when class switching takes place. So by arranging to have appropriate cytokines produced at the appropriate places, Mother Nature can insure that the right class of antibody is made to defend against a particular invader.

The other change that can take place as a B cell matures is somatic hypermutation. In contrast to class switching, in which the antibody gets a different Fc region, somatic hypermutation alters the antigen-binding region of the antibody. Because the probability that a B cell will proliferate depends on the affinity of its BCR for antigen, the B cells that proliferate most will be those for which somatic hypermutation has increased the binding affinity of their BCRs. Consequently, somatic hypermutation and selection for proliferation result in a collection of B cells whose BCRs, on average, bind more tightly to the invader than did the original, unmutated BCRs. These upgraded B cells are especially useful as memory cells. Because their affinity-matured BCRs are sensitive to small amounts of antigen, these B cells can be reactivated early in a second infection while the number of invaders is still relatively small.

B cells can be activated with or without T cell help, but the outcomes in these two cases usually are very different. T cell-independent activation generally results in the production of IgM antibodies. In contrast, T cell-dependent activation can result in affinity matured, IgG, IgA, or IgE antibodies. One reason for this difference is that both class switching and somatic hypermutation require ligation of CD40 proteins on B cells. This signal is usually provided by CD40L, a protein found on the surface of activated helper T cells.

As B cells mature, they must decide whether to become short-lived plasma cells, which produce vast quantities of antibodies, or to stick around as longer lived memory B cells. These memory B cells are responsible for making the antibodies which can protect us from a subsequent attack by the same pathogen.

SUMMARY FIGURE

Our summary figure now includes the innate immune system from the last lecture plus B cells and antibodies.

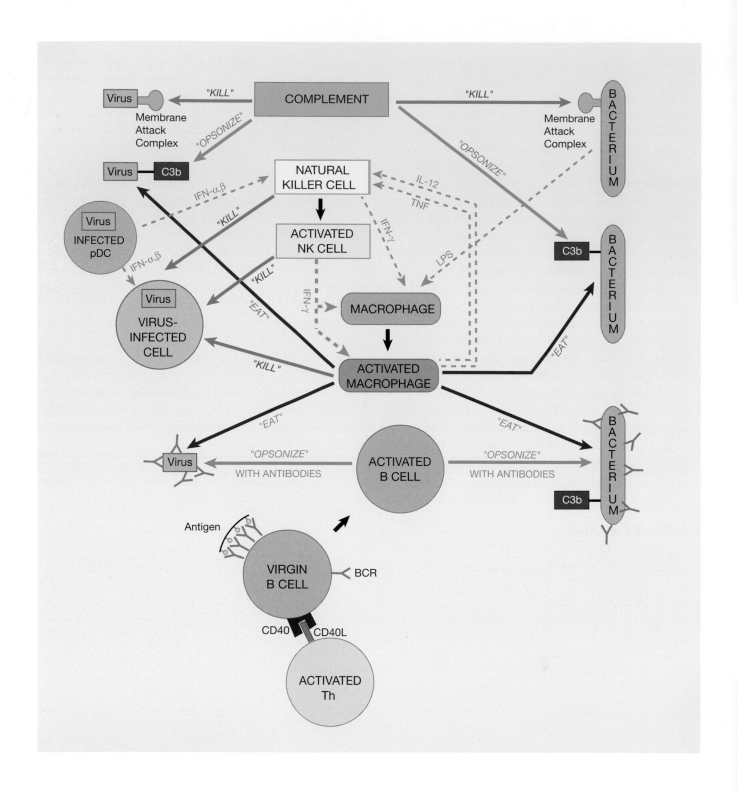

THOUGHT QUESTIONS

1. B cells are produced according to the principle of clonal selection. Exactly what does this mean?

2. Describe what happens during T cell-dependent activation of B cells.

3. How can B cells be activated without T cell help, and why is T cell-independent activation of B cells important in defending us against certain pathogens?

4. Describe fail-safe systems that are involved in B cell activation.

5. What are the main attributes of IgM, IgG, IgA, and IgE antibodies?

6. Why do class switching and somatic hypermutation produce B cells that are better able to defend against invaders?

7. What is the difference between co-stimulation and co-activation?

LECTURE 4

The Magic of Antigen Presentation

HEADS UP!

For T cells to be activated, their receptors must recognize protein fragments presented by MHC molecules on the surface of special "antigen presenting cells." Presentation of antigen by class I MHC molecules lets killer T cells "look into" cells to determine if they are infected and should be destroyed. Presentation of antigen by class II MHC molecules helps guarantee that the decision to deploy the powerful adaptive immune system is not made by a single cell. Within the human population, there are genes for many, slightly different MHC molecules. Consequently, it is likely that at least some humans will have MHC molecules which can display protein fragments from any pathogen.

INTRODUCTION

Of all the concepts on which the immune system is based, perhaps the most elegant, and certainly the most unexpected, is antigen presentation: the concept of having one cell present protein fragments to another cell. As you will see, antigen presentation is central to the function of the adaptive immune system, with the cells that present antigen to T cells – the **antigen presenting cells (APCs)** – playing a pivotal role. Let's begin by discussing the "billboards" on APCs that actually do the presenting: the class I and class II MHC molecules.

CLASS I MHC MOLECULES

The structures of class I and class II MHC molecules have now been carefully analyzed, so we have a good idea what both kinds of molecules look like. Class I molecules have a binding groove that is closed at both ends, so the small protein fragments (**peptides**) they present must fit within the confines of the groove (the "bun," if you will). Indeed, **when immunologists pried peptides from the grasp of class I molecules and sequenced them, they found that most of them are eight or nine amino acids in length. These peptides are anchored at the ends, and the slight variation in length is accommodated by letting the peptide bulge out a bit in the center.**

Every human has three genes (**HLA-A, HLA-B, and HLA-C**) for class I MHC proteins on chromosome 6. Because we have two chromosome 6's (one from Mom and one from Dad), we all have a total of six class I MHC genes. Each class I HLA protein pairs with another protein called **β2-microglobulin** to make up the complete class I MHC molecule. In the human population, there are about 1500 slightly different forms of the genes that encode the three class I HLA proteins. The proteins encoded by the variants of the HLA-A, HLA-B, and HLA-C genes have roughly the same shape, but they differ by one or a few amino acids. Immunologists call molecules that have many forms "polymorphic," and the class I HLA proteins certainly fit this description. In contrast, all of us have the same gene for the β2-microglobulin protein.

Because they are polymorphic, class I MHC molecules can have different binding motifs, and therefore can present peptides which have different kinds of amino acids at their ends. For example, some class I MHC molecules bind to peptides that have hydrophobic amino acids at one end, whereas other MHC molecules prefer basic amino acids at this anchor position. Since humans have the possibility of expressing up to six different class I molecules, collectively our class I molecules can present a wide variety of peptides. Moreover, although MHC I molecules are picky about binding to certain amino acids at the ends of the peptide, they are rather promiscuous in their selection of amino acids at the center of the protein fragment.

How the Immune System Works, Fifth Edition. Lauren Sompayrac. © 2016 John Wiley & Sons, Ltd. Published 2016 by John Wiley & Sons, Ltd.

As a result, a given class I MHC molecule can bind to and present a large number of different peptides, each of which "fits" with the particular amino acids present at the ends of its binding groove.

CLASS II MHC MOLECULES

Like class I molecules, the class II MHC molecules (encoded by genes in the HLA-D region of chromosome 6) are wildly polymorphic. Within the human population, there are about 700 different versions of the class II MHC molecules. In contrast to class I MHC molecules, the binding groove of class II MHC molecules is open at both ends, so a peptide can hang out of the groove. As you might expect from this feature, peptides that bind to class II molecules are longer than those that occupy the closed groove of class I molecules – in the range of 13–25 amino acids. Further, for class II MHC molecules, the critical amino acids that anchor the peptides are spaced along the binding groove instead of being clustered at the ends.

ANTIGEN PRESENTATION BY CLASS I MHC MOLECULES

MHC I molecules are billboards that display on the surface of a cell, fragments of proteins manufactured by that cell. Immunologists call these **endogenous proteins**. These include ordinary cellular proteins like enzymes and structural proteins, as well as proteins encoded by viruses and other parasites that may have infected the cell. For example, when a virus enters a cell, it uses the cellular biosynthetic machinery to produce proteins encoded by viral genes. A sample of these viral proteins is then displayed by class I MHC molecules along with samples of all the normal cellular proteins. So in effect, the MHC I billboards advertise a sample of all the proteins that are being made inside a cell. Almost every cell in the human body expresses class I molecules on its surface, although the number of molecules varies from cell to cell. Killer T cells (also called cytotoxic lymphocytes or CTLs) inspect the protein fragments displayed by class I MHC molecules. Consequently, almost every cell is an "open book" that can be checked by CTLs to determine whether it has been invaded by a virus or other parasite and should be destroyed. Importantly, after they have been on the surface for a short while, the MHC billboards are replaced by new ones – so the class I MHC display is kept current.

The way endogenous proteins are processed and loaded onto class I MHC molecules is very interesting. When mRNA is translated into protein in the cytoplasm of a cell, mistakes are frequently made. These mistakes can result in the production of useless proteins that don't fold up correctly. In addition, proteins suffer damage due to normal wear and tear. So to make sure our cells don't fill up with defective proteins, old or useless proteins are rapidly fed into protein-destroying "machines" in the cytoplasm that function rather like wood chippers. These protein chippers are called **proteasomes**, and they cut proteins up into peptides. Most of these peptides are then broken down further into individual amino acids, which are reused to make new proteins. However, some of the peptides created by the proteasomes are carried by specific transporter proteins (**TAP1** and **TAP2**) across the membrane of the **endoplasmic reticulum (ER)** – a large, sack-like structure inside the cell from which most proteins destined for transport to the cell surface begin their journey.

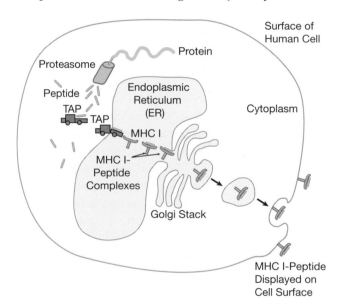

Once inside the ER, some peptides are chosen to be loaded into the grooves of class I MHC molecules. I say "chosen," because, as we discussed, not all peptides will fit. For starters, a peptide must be the right length – about nine amino acids. In addition, the amino acids at the ends of the peptide must be compatible with the anchor amino acids that line the ends of the groove of the MHC molecule. Obviously, not all of the "chips" prepared by the proteasome will have these characteristics, and those that don't are degraded or shipped back out of the ER into the cytoplasm. Once class I MHC molecules are loaded with peptides, they proceed to the surface of the cell for display. So there are three main steps in preparing a class I display: generation of a peptide by the proteasome, transport of the peptide into the ER by the TAP transporter, and binding of the peptide to the groove of the MHC I molecule.

In "ordinary" cells like liver cells and heart cells, the major function of proteasomes is to deal with defective proteins. So as you can imagine, the chippers in these cells are not too particular about how proteins are cut up – they just hack away. As a result, some of the peptides will be appropriate for MHC presentation, but most will not be. In contrast, in cells like macrophages that specialize in presenting antigen, this chipping is not so random. For example, binding of IFN-γ to receptors on the surface of a macrophage upregulates expression of three proteins called LMP2, LMP7, and MECL1. These proteins replace three "stock" proteins which are part of the normal proteasome machinery. The result of this replacement is that the "customized" proteasomes now preferentially cut proteins after hydrophobic or basic amino acids. Why, you ask? Because the TAP transporter and MHC I molecules both favor peptides that have either hydrophobic or basic C-termini. So in antigen presenting cells, standard proteasomes are modified so they will produce custom-made peptides, thereby increasing the efficiency of class I display.

Proteasomes also are not too particular about the size of peptides they make, and since the magic number for class I presentation is about nine amino acids, you might imagine that the ER would be flooded with useless peptides that are either too long or too short. However, it turns out that the TAP transporter has the highest affinity for peptides that are 8–16 amino acids long. Consequently, the TAP transporter screens peptides produced by proteasomes, and preferentially transports those that have the right kinds of C-termini and which are approximately the correct length. Once candidate peptides have been transported into the ER, enzymes then trim off excess N-terminal amino acids to make the peptide the right size for binding to class I MHC molecules.

An important feature of this "chop it up and present it" system is that the majority of the proteins chopped up by proteasomes are newly synthesized proteins which are structurally flawed. In fact, it is estimated that about half of all proteins produced by the cell are defective. Consequently, most proteins are displayed on class I MHC molecules soon after they are produced. This means that you don't have to wait for proteins to wear out before they can be chopped up and presented – making it possible for the immune system to react quickly to an infection.

ANTIGEN PRESENTATION BY CLASS II MHC MOLECULES

Whereas class I MHC molecules are designed to present protein fragments to killer T cells, class II MHC molecules present peptides to helper T cells. And in contrast to class I MHC molecules, which are expressed on almost every kind of cell, class II molecules are expressed exclusively on cells of the immune system. This makes sense. Class I molecules specialize in displaying proteins that are manufactured inside the cell, so the ubiquity of class I molecules gives CTLs a chance to check most cells in the body for infection. On the other hand, class II MHC molecules function as billboards that advertise what is happening outside the cell to alert helper T cells to danger. Therefore, relatively few cells expressing class II are required for this task – just enough to sample the environment in various parts of the body.

The two proteins that make up the class II MHC molecules (called the α and β chains) are produced in the cytoplasm and are injected into the endoplasmic reticulum where they bind to a third protein called the **invariant chain**. This invariant chain protein performs several functions. First, it sits in the groove of the MHC II molecule and keeps it from picking up other peptides in the ER. This is important, because the ER is full of endogenous peptides that have been processed by proteasomes for loading onto class I MHC molecules. If these protein fragments were loaded onto class II molecules, then class I and class II MHC molecules would display the same kind of peptides: those made from proteins produced in the cell. Since the goal is for class II MHC molecules to present antigens that come from outside the cell, the **exogenous proteins**, the invariant chain performs an important function by acting as a "chaperone" that makes sure "inappropriate suitors" (endogenous peptides) don't get picked up by MHC II molecules in the ER.

Another function of the invariant chain is to guide class II MHC molecules out through the Golgi stack to special vesicles in the cytoplasm called **endosomes**. It is within endosomes that class II MHC molecules are loaded with peptides. The current thinking is that while class II MHC molecules are making their way from the ER to an endosome, proteins that are hanging around outside the cell are enclosed in a phagosome, and brought into the cell. This phagosome then merges with the endosome, and enzymes present in the endosome chop up the exogenous proteins into peptides. During this time, endosomal enzymes also destroy all of the invariant chain except for the piece called **CLIP** that actually is guarding the groove of the MHC molecule. Amazingly, although the exogenous proteins and the invariant chain are hacked to pieces by enzymes in the endosome, the class II MHC molecule itself remains unscathed. This is presumably because the MHC molecule is cleverly folded so that the enzymes cannot gain access to their favorite cleavage sites.

Meanwhile, a cellular protein, **HLA-DM**, which also has traveled to the endosome, catalyzes the release of CLIP, allowing an exogenous peptide to be loaded into the now-empty groove of the class II MHC molecule. But HLA-DM does more than just kick CLIP out to make room for the peptide. HLA-DM competes with potential peptides for binding to the class II MHC molecule, insuring that only peptides that bind tightly will be presented. Finally, the complex of MHC plus peptide is transported to the cell surface for display.

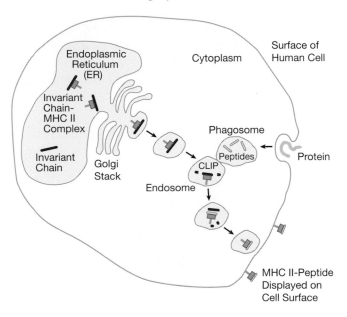

It is important to recognize that there are two separate loading sites and pathways for class I and class II MHC molecules. It is this separation of loading sites and pathways that allows the class I billboard to advertise what's going on inside the cell (for killer T cells), and the class II billboard to advertise what's happening outside (for helper T cells).

ANTIGEN PRESENTING CELLS

Before a killer T cell can kill or a helper T cell can help, it must be activated. For this to happen, a T cell must recognize its cognate antigen presented by an MHC molecule on the surface of another cell. But this is not enough. It must also receive a second, co-stimulatory signal. Only certain cells are equipped to provide both class I and class II MHC display and co-stimulation. These are the **antigen presenting cells (APCs)**.

Because the job of APCs is to activate killer and helper T cells, these cells really should have been named "T cell-activating cells." This would have avoided confusion with the "ordinary" cells in the body, which cannot activate T cells, but which do use class I MHC molecules to present antigens made inside these cells to alert killer T cells. Does it seem to you that immunologists just like to make things confusing? I sometimes think so. Anyway, to keep this straight, just remember that the term "antigen presenting cell" always refers to those special cells which can provide both the high levels of MHC proteins and co-stimulatory molecules required for T cell activation.

Co-stimulation usually involves a protein called **B7** on the surface of an antigen presenting cell that "plugs into" a protein called **CD28** on the surface of a T cell.

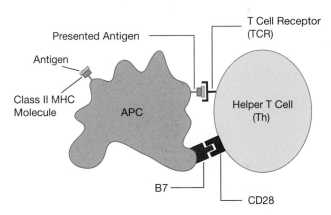

Three types of antigen presenting cells have been identified: activated dendritic cells, activated macrophages, and activated B cells. It's interesting that all of these are white blood cells which start life in the bone marrow, migrate out to various sites in the body, and then must be activated before they can function as antigen presenting cells. New blood cells are made continuously, so APCs can be replenished as needed.

Activated dendritic cells

Dendritic cells (DCs) have a characteristic, starfish-like shape, and get their name from the word "dendrite," which is commonly used to describe the projections on nerve cells. It is important to note that these cells are very different from the plasmacytoid dendritic cells (pDCs) mentioned earlier – cells whose primary function is to produce large amounts of interferon α and β in response to a viral attack. In fact, pDCs are not even shaped like a starfish. They are round, like plasma cells.

Dendritic cells once were considered to be only a curiosity. However, it is now appreciated that these cells are the most important of all the antigen presenting cells – because **dendritic cells can initiate the immune response by activating** virgin **T cells.** Here's how this works.

The first DCs described were starfish-shaped, "Langerhans" cells that are found in the tissues just below the skin. However, dendritic cells have since been discovered all over the body. What is now clear is that these dendritic cells are "sentinel" cells which take up positions beneath the barriers of epithelial cells that represent our first line of defense. In normal tissues (tissues that have not been infected), DCs resemble wine tasters. Although they can take up about four times their volume of extracellular fluid per hour, they mostly just take it in and spit it back out. In this "resting" state, DCs express some B7 and relatively low levels of MHC molecules on their surface. As a result, these resting dendritic cells are not very good at presenting antigen to T cells, especially to virgin T cells. This is because **naive T cells require extensive receptor crosslinking by MHC–peptide complexes as well as powerful co-stimulation in order to be activated.**

If there is a microbial invasion, and the tissues in which a dendritic cell resides become a battleground, the dendritic cell will become "activated." DCs can be activated by signals which come from other immune system cells that are engaged in battle. For example, both neutrophils and macrophages give off tumor necrosis factor (TNF) when they are trying to destroy an attacker, and this battle cytokine can activate DCs. Also, cells that are being killed by invaders give off chemicals that can result in DC activation. Finally, dendritic cells have pattern-recognition receptors (e.g., Toll-like receptors) which they use to recognize molecular patterns that are characteristic of broad classes of invaders. The signals received by these pattern-recognition receptors can play an important role in activating dendritic cells.

Dendritic cells travel

When a dendritic cell is activated by battle cytokines, chemicals given off by dying cells, ligation of its pattern-recognition receptors, or a combination of these signals, the lifestyle of this "wine taster" changes dramatically. No longer does the dendritic cell "sip and spit." Now it "swallows" what it has taken in. Typically, a DC remains in the tissues for about 6 hours after activation, collecting a representa-

tive sample of battle antigens. At that point, phagocytosis ceases, and the activated dendritic cell leaves the tissues and travels through the lymphatic system to the nearest lymph node. **It is its ability to "travel when activated" that makes the dendritic antigen presenting cell so special.**

Inside a resting DC are large numbers of "reserve" class II MHC molecules. When a resting DC is activated and starts to "mature," these class II MHC molecules begin to be loaded with antigens from the battle scene. And by the time a DC reaches its destination – a trip that usually takes about a day – these battle antigen-loaded class II MHC molecules will be prominently displayed on the surface of the cell. Also during its journey, the DC upregulates expression of its class I MHC molecules. Consequently, if the dendritic cell had been infected by a virus out at the battle scene, by the time it reaches a lymph node, fragments of viral proteins will be on display on the dendritic cell's class I MHC billboards. Finally, while traveling, the DC increases production of B7 co-stimulatory proteins. So **when it reaches a lymph node, the mature dendritic cell has everything it needs to activate virgin T cells: high levels of class I and class II MHC molecules loaded with the appropriate peptides, and plenty of B7 proteins.**

Three Phases in the Life of a Dendritic Cell

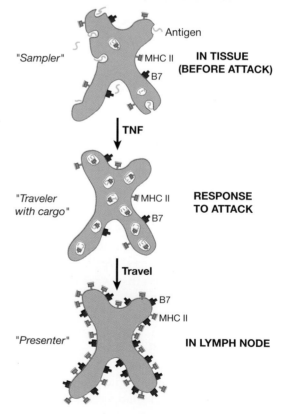

Now, why do you think DCs, which wildly sample antigens out in the tissues, stop their sampling when they begin their journey to a lymph node? Of course. Dendritic cells take a "snapshot" of what is happening on the "front lines," and carry this image to a lymph node – the place where virgin T cells congregate. There the traveling dendritic cells activate those virgin T cells whose T cell receptors recognize the invader that is "in the picture." The fact that battle cytokines such as TNF trigger the migration of DCs to a lymph node also makes perfect sense. After all, you want DCs to mature, travel to lymph nodes, and present antigen only if a battle is on.

Once a DC reaches a lymph node, it only lives for about a week. This short lifetime may seem strange at first. After all, this doesn't give a dendritic cell very long to meet up with the "right" virgin T cell which is circulating through the lymph nodes, looking for its cognate antigen. However, dendritic cells can interact with hundreds or even thousands of T cells every hour, and their short presentation life insures that dendritic cells carry snapshots of the battle which are up-to-date. In addition, after a dendritic cell has been activated, but before it begins its travels, it produces special cytokines (chemokines) which encourage white blood cells called **monocytes** to leave the blood, enter the tissues, and become dendritic cells. Consequently, **activated dendritic cells recruit their own replacements**. These newly recruited DCs can carry fresh images of the battle to lymph nodes as the battle continues.

There is another reason for the short lifetime of dendritic cells. In Lecture 2, I mentioned that it is very important that the magnitude of an immune response be in proportion to the seriousness of the attack. The short lifetime of DCs helps make this happen. Here's how.

During a microbial attack, the number of T cells activated will depend on the number of mature dendritic cells that bring news of the battle to nearby lymph nodes. If the attack is weak, relatively few battle cytokines will be produced by warring macrophages, and only a small number of dendritic cells will be dispatched with their cargo. And because these DCs only live a short time once they reach the lymph node, only a limited number of T cells will be activated – just enough to deal with the small number of microbial invaders. On the other hand, if the infection is serious, many battle cytokines will be produced, many dendritic cells will be activated and travel to nearby lymph nodes, many more DCs will be recruited from the blood, and many T cells will be activated. Consequently, one result of the dendritic cell's short lifetime is that the number of DCs in the lymph nodes at a given moment will reflect the current situation at the battle site, and the magnitude of the immune response will be in proportion to the severity of the infection.

So dendritic antigen presenting cells are sentinel cells that "sample" antigens out in the tissues. If there is an invasion, DCs become activated and travel to nearby lymph nodes. There they initiate the adaptive immune response by presenting antigen collected at the battle scene to virgin T cells. Activated DCs are short-lived, and the rapid turnover of these cells insures that the "pictures" they bring to a lymph node are continuously updated. Moreover, the number of dendritic cells dispatched from the tissues and the number of replacement dendritic cells recruited will depend on the severity of the attack. Consequently, the immune system is able to mount a response that is proportional to the danger posed by the invasion. Can you imagine a more ingenious system? I don't think so!

Dendritic cells are classified as part of the innate immune system because their receptors are "hard-wired" and not "adaptable" like those of B and T cells. However, as I'm sure you now understand, DCs actually function as a "bridge" between the innate and the adaptive systems.

Activated macrophages

Macrophages also are sentinel cells which stand guard over areas of our body that are exposed to the outside world. They are very adaptable cells which can function as garbage collectors, antigen presenting cells, or ferocious killers – depending on the signals they receive from the microenvironment in which they reside. In a resting state, macrophages are good at tidying up, but they are not much good at antigen presentation. This is because macrophages only express enough MHC and co-stimulatory molecules to function as antigen presenting cells after they have been activated by battle cytokines such as IFN-γ, or by having their pattern-recognition receptors (e.g., their Toll-like receptors) ligated by invading pathogens.

So macrophages resemble dendritic cells in that they efficiently present antigen only when there is something dangerous to present. However, it is important to recognize that **dendritic antigen presenting cells don't kill, and macrophages don't travel**. Indeed, DCs can be pictured as "photojournalists" who don't carry weapons, who take snapshots of the fighting, and who then leave the battlefield to file their stories. In contrast, macrophages are heavily armed soldiers who must stand and fight. After all, macrophages are one of our main weapons in the early defense against invaders. Nevertheless, their lack of mobility raises an interesting question: What good is the activated macrophage's capacity to present antigen if it can't travel to lymph nodes where virgin T cells are located? Here's the answer.

Once they have been activated by dendritic cells, T cells exit the lymph nodes, circulate through the blood, and enter inflamed tissues to help with the battle. However, these "experienced" T cells must be continually re-stimulated. Otherwise, they think the battle has been won, and they go back to a resting state or die of neglect. That's where activated macrophages come in. Macrophages act as "refueling stations" which keep experienced T cells "turned on" so they can continue to participate in the battle. So **mature dendritic cells activate virgin T cells, and activated macrophages mainly function to re-stimulate experienced T cells**.

Activated B cells

The third APC is the activated B cell. A virgin B cell is not much good at antigen presentation, because it expresses only low levels of class II MHC molecules and little or no B7. However, once a B cell has been activated, the levels of class II MHC molecules and B7 proteins on its surface increase dramatically. As a result, an experienced **B cell is able to act as an antigen presenting cell for Th cells.** B cells are not used as APCs during the initial stages of an infection, because at that time they are still naive – they haven't been activated. However, later in the course of the infection or during subsequent infections, presentation of antigen by experienced B cells plays an important role. This is because B cells have one great advantage over the other APCs: **B cells can concentrate antigen for presentation.** After a B cell's receptors have bound to their cognate antigen, the whole complex of BCR plus antigen is removed from the cell surface and dragged into the cell. There the antigen is processed, loaded onto class II MHC molecules, and transported back to the cell surface for presentation.

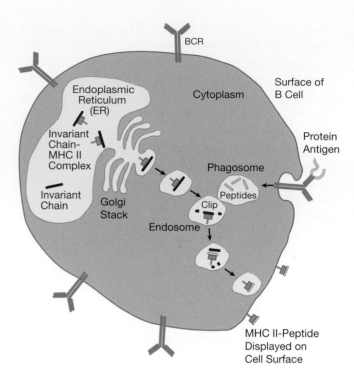

Because B cell receptors have such a high affinity for antigen, they act like "magnets," collecting antigen for presentation to Th cells. Since a threshold number of T cell receptors must be crosslinked by presented antigen before a Th cell can be activated, it is estimated that activated B cells have a 100- to 10 000-fold advantage over other APCs in activating helper T cells at times when there is relatively little antigen around. Presentation of antigen by B cells is also very fast. Less than half an hour elapses between the time antigen is captured by a B cell's receptors and the time it is displayed on the cell surface by class II MHC molecules.

In summary, **when an invader is first encountered, all the B cells which could recognize that particular invader are virgins, so the important APCs are activated dendritic cells. Then, while the battle is raging, activated macrophages on the front lines present antigen to warring T cells to keep them pumped up. Later in the infection, or if this same invader is encountered again, experienced B cells are extremely important APCs – because they can quickly activate helper T cells by concentrating small amounts of antigen for presentation.**

THE LOGIC OF CLASS I MHC PRESENTATION

To really appreciate why antigen presentation is one of Mother Nature's greatest "inventions," we need to think a little about the logic behind this amazing activity. For starters, we need to ask the question: Why bother with MHC presentation at all? Why not just let a T cell's receptors recognize un-presented antigen the way a B cell's receptors do? This is really a two-part question, since we are talking about two rather different displays: class I and class II. So let's examine these one at a time.

Certainly one reason for class I presentation is to focus the attention of killer T cells on infected cells, not on viruses and other pathogens that are outside our cells in the blood and tissues. So long as pathogens remain outside of our cells, antibodies can tag them for destruction by professional phagocytes, and can bind to them and prevent them from initiating an infection. Since each plasma B cell can pump out about 2000 antibody molecules per second, these antibodies are "cheap" weapons that deal quite effectively with extracellular invaders. However, once microbes enter a cell, antibodies can't get at them. When this happens, killer T cells – the high-tech, "expensive" weapons, specifically designed to destroy infected cells – are needed. And the requirement that killer T cells recognize antigens presented by class I MHC molecules on infected cells insures that CTLs won't waste their time going after invaders that are outside of cells – invaders which antibodies usually can deal with quite effectively.

In addition, it would be extremely dangerous to have un-presented antigen signal T cell killing. Imagine how terrible it would be if uninfected cells happened to have debris from dead viruses stuck to their surfaces, and killer T cells recognized this un-presented antigen and killed these "innocent bystander" cells. That certainly wouldn't do.

Another reason class I display is so important is that most proteins made in a pathogen-infected cell remain inside the cell, and never make their way to the cell surface. So without class I display, many pathogen-infected cells would go undetected by killer T cells. In fact, part of the magic of the class I MHC display is that, in principle, every protein of an invading pathogen can be chopped up and displayed by class I MHC molecules for killer T cells to view.

Finally, because their receptors recognize "native" antigens that have not been fragmented and presented, B cells actually are at a disadvantage. The reason is that most proteins must be folded in order to function properly. As a result of this folding, many epitopes that a B cell's receptors might recognize are unavailable for viewing – because they are on the inside of a folded protein molecule. In contrast, when a protein is chopped up into short pieces and presented by class I MHC molecules, epitopes cannot be hidden from killer T cells.

So the logic of class I MHC presentation is easy to understand, but why did Mother Nature make MHC molecules so polymorphic? After all, there are so many different forms in the human population that most of us inherit genes for six different class I molecules. Doesn't this seem a bit excessive?

Well, suppose there were only a few different class I MHC proteins. Now imagine what might happen if a virus were to mutate so that none of its peptides would bind to any of these MHC I molecules. Such a virus might wipe out the entire human population, because no killer T cells could be activated to destroy virus-infected cells. So polymorphic MHC molecules give at least some people in the population a chance of surviving an attack by a clever pathogen.

Okay, but why does each of us have six genes for class I MHC proteins? That seems like a lot, especially since the class I MHC proteins are so polymorphic. The answer is that the possibility of "owning" up to six different class I MHC molecules increases the probability that each of us, individually, will have at least one class I MHC molecule into which a given pathogen's protein fragments will fit. Indeed, AIDS patients who have inherited the maximum number of different class I MHC molecules (six) live significantly longer than patients who have genes encoding only five or fewer different class I molecules. The thinking here is that as the AIDS virus mutates, having a larger number of different class I molecules increases the probability that mutated viral proteins can be presented. Why six, not ten, genes for class I MHC molecules? Beats me!

THE LOGIC OF CLASS II MHC PRESENTATION

Okay, so class I MHC presentation makes a lot of sense. But what about class II presentation? At first glance, this "dual display" (class I and class II) by antigen presenting cells might seem overly complicated. What must be appreciated, however, is that many pathogens do not infect human cells: They are quite happy living and reproducing outside our cells in our tissues or in our blood. If antigen presenting cells could only display proteins made by pathogens that infect them, intelligence on many of the most dangerous microbes would never reach the command centers in lymph nodes. By using class II MHC molecules to advertise a sampling of the total environment at the battle front, intelligence on all types of invaders can be made available to helper T cells.

But couldn't helper T cells just recognize un-presented antigen? After all, they aren't killers, so there isn't the problem of bystander killing. That's true, of course, but there is still a safety issue here. Antigen presenting cells only present antigen efficiently when a battle is going on, and helper T cells are educated not to react against our own proteins. Consequently, both the helper T cell and the antigen presenting cell must "agree" that there has been an invasion before a helper T cell can be activated. By requiring that helper T cells only recognize presented antigen, Mother Nature guarantees that the decision to deploy the potentially deadly adaptive immune system is not made by a single cell.

Also, like class I molecules, class II molecules present small fragments of proteins. As a result, the number of targets that a helper T cell can "see" during presentation far exceeds those available for viewing in a large, folded protein. The consequence of this expanded number of targets is a stronger, more diverse immune reaction in which many different helper T cells will be activated – helper T cells whose receptors recognize the many different epitopes that make up the antigens of an invader.

CROSS-PRESENTATION

Although the separation of class I and class II pathways is the "law," it has been shown that a certain subset of antigen presenting cells can take up exogenous antigens and shuttle them into the class I pathway for presentation by class I MHC molecules. Such an unlawful use of the class I display has been termed **cross-presentation**. The idea is that if a clever pathogen (e.g., a virus) figured out a way to avoid infecting antigen presenting cells, yet could still infect and reproduce in other cells of the body, cross-presentation would give the immune system a chance to activate CTLs against this pathogen. So far, the rules that govern cross-presentation have not been clearly defined. Moreover, it is not yet known whether, under normal

circumstances, cross-presentation is an important feature of the human immune system.

NON-CLASSICAL MHC MOLECULES AND LIPID PRESENTATION

Class I and class II MHC molecules are called classical MHC molecules. So as you might expect, there also are non-classical MHC molecules. The best studied of these is the CD1 family of proteins. These non-classical MHC molecules resemble class I MHC molecules in that they consist of a long, heavy chain protein which is paired with the β2-microglobulin protein. However, in contrast to classical MHC molecules, which have grooves that are suitable to bind short peptides, the CD1, non-classical MHC molecules have grooves which are designed to bind lipids. CD1 molecules can "sample" lipids from various compartments within a cell, and can present these molecules on the surface of antigen presenting cells, where they can activate T cells. Consequently, it has been postulated that these non-classical MHC molecules give T cells a way of surveying the lipid composition of cells, just as class I MHC molecules allow T cells to examine a cell's proteins.

For every rule in immunology there seems to be an exception, and the rule has been that T cells only recognize fragments of proteins presented by class I and class II MHC molecules. Obviously, CD1 presentation of lipids to T cells is an exception to this rule. So far, however, it is not clear how important lipid presentation is for the immune defense. Consequently, I will "stick to the rule" that T cells only recognize protein antigens. Be aware, however, that this may change as more research is done on CD1-presented lipids.

MHC PROTEINS AND ORGAN TRANSPLANTS

In addition to their "natural" role in antigen presentation, MHC molecules also are important in the "unnatural" setting of organ and tissue transplantation. Transplantation studies actually began in the 1930s with experiments involving mouse tumors. In those days, tumors were usually induced by rubbing some horrible chemical on the skin of a mouse, and then waiting for a long time for a tumor to develop. Because it was so much trouble to make these tumors, biologists wanted to keep the tumor cells alive for study after the mouse had died. They did this by injecting some of the tumor cells into another, healthy mouse, where the cells would continue to grow. What they observed, however, was that the tumor cells only could be successfully transplanted when the two mice were from a strain of mice in which there had been a lot of inbreeding. And the more inbred the strain, the better the chance for survival of the transplant. This provided the impetus for the creation of a number of inbred mouse strains that immunologists depend on today. Just so you know, it takes over two years of constant breeding to produce a strain of mice that is truly inbred – a strain in which all the mice have essentially the same genetic makeup.

Once inbred mouse strains were available, immunologists began to study the transplantation of normal tissues from one mouse to another. Right away they noticed that if a small patch of skin from one mouse was grafted onto the skin of another mouse, this new skin retained its healthy pink color and continued to grow – so long as the two mice were from the same inbred strain. In contrast, when this experiment was tried with mice that were not inbred, the transplanted skin turned white within hours (because the blood supply had been cut off) and invariably died. Immunologists figured this immediate graft rejection must be due to some genetic incompatibility, because it did not occur with inbred mice that have the same genes. To identify the genes that are involved in "tissue compatibility" (**histocompatibility**), immunologists bred mice to create strains that differed by only a few genes, yet which were still incompatible for tissue transplants. Whenever they did these experiments, they kept identifying genes that were grouped in a complex on mouse chromosome 17 – a complex they eventually called the "major histocompatibility complex" or MHC.

So **the MHC molecules that we have been discussing in the context of antigen presentation are the very same molecules that are responsible for immediate rejection of transplanted organs.** It turns out that killer T cells are particularly sensitive to MHC molecules that are "foreign," and when they see them, they attack and kill the cells that express them. Some of their favorite targets are the cells that make up the blood vessels contained within the donated organ. By destroying these vessels, CTLs cut off the blood supply to the transplanted organ, usually resulting in its death. For this reason, transplant surgeons try to match donors and recipients who have the same MHC molecules. However, finding such a match is difficult. Indeed, it is estimated that if you had access to organs contributed by 10 000 000 different individuals who were not related to you, the chance of your finding an exact match to all your class I and class II MHC molecules would only be about 50%. So the diversity of MHC molecules, which is so important in protecting us from new or mutated invaders, creates a real problem for organ transplantation. Clearly, the immune system did not evolve with organ swapping in mind!

REVIEW

Class I MHC molecules function as billboards that display what is going on inside a cell. For example, when a virus infects a cell, it uses that cell's biosynthetic machinery to produce viral proteins. Some of these proteins are cut up into small pieces (peptides) by the proteasome, and carried by the TAP transporters into the endoplasmic reticulum (ER). There the peptides are "interviewed" by class I molecules. Those that are about nine amino acids in length with appropriate amino acids at their ends are bound in the grooves of class I MHC molecules, and are transported to the surface of the cell. By scanning the MHC I–peptide complexes displayed there, killer T cells can "look into a cell" to determine whether it has been infected and should be destroyed.

Class II MHC molecules also are billboards, but they are designed to alert helper T cells that a battle is being waged. Class II molecules are assembled in the ER, just like class I molecules, but because invariant chain proteins occupy their binding grooves, class II molecules do not pick up peptides in the ER. Instead, the class II-invariant chain complex is transported out of the ER and into another cellular compartment called an endosome. There they meet up with proteins that have been taken into the cell by phagocytosis and cut up into peptides by enzymes. These peptides then replace the invariant chains that have been guarding the grooves of the class II molecules, and the MHC–peptide complexes are transported to the cell surface for display to Th cells.

By this clever mechanism, class II molecules pick up peptides derived from proteins taken in from outside the cell, but avoid peptides derived from proteins made within the cell.

The display by MHC molecules of fragmented proteins has several advantages over a display of intact proteins. First, most viral proteins normally remain hidden inside an infected cell and are not found on the cell surface. Therefore, these proteins would never be seen by killer T cells unless they were advertised by class I MHC molecules. In addition, because protein folding can hide large portions of a protein from view, chopping a protein up into small peptides reveals many potential T cell targets that would be inaccessible in an intact protein. Consequently, MHC display greatly increases the probability that CTLs will recognize an infected cell, and that helper T cells will be alerted to a microbial attack.

Both class I and class II MHC molecules are extremely polymorphic, and humans have multiple genes for both classes of MHC molecules. Consequently, it is likely that your MHC molecules will be able to display peptides from most pathogens, and that at least some people in the population will have MHC molecules capable of displaying peptides from any pathogen.

Antigen presenting cells are special immune system cells that can provide both class I and class II MHC display as well as co-stimulation. The most important antigen presenting cell during the initial stages of an attack is the dendritic cell, because this cell can activate virgin T cells. When a DC detects danger signals at the scene of the battle, it begins to mature, and migrates with its cargo of "battle antigen" to a nearby lymph node. There, the dendritic cell uses class II MHC molecules to display fragments of proteins it has collected out in the tissues, and class I MHC molecules to display fragments of proteins made by viruses or bacteria that may have infected the dendritic cell out at the battle site. In this way, the dendritic cell effectively takes a snapshot of what is going on at the front, carries it to the place where T cells are plentiful, and then does its "show and tell" thing to activate T cells.

Macrophages, activated by danger signals, also can function as antigen presenting cells. However, activated macrophages don't travel to lymph nodes to present antigen. They stay put in the tissues and battle invaders. Consequently, macrophages are most useful for presenting antigen after the adaptive immune system has been activated. At that time, activated macrophages out in the tissues can keep experienced T cells fired up, prolonging the time that they are effective in dealing with invaders.

Activated B cells are the third type of antigen presenting cell, but again, these cells aren't useful in initiating the adaptive response against a new invader. The reason is that before B cells can function as antigen presenting cells, they must first be activated by helper T cells – and Th cells must wait to be activated by dendritic cells. So B cells don't get "certified" to be antigen presenting cells until after the adaptive immune response has already fired up. Nevertheless, once activated, B cells have a great advantage over DCs and macrophages: B cells can use their receptors as "antigen collectors" to concentrate small amounts of antigen for presentation to helper T cells. Consequently, relatively late in the initial infection or early in a subsequent infection by the same attacker, B cells play a major role as antigen presenting cells.

SUMMARY FIGURE

You will notice that our summary figure now includes antigen presenting cells with their MHC and B7 molecules.

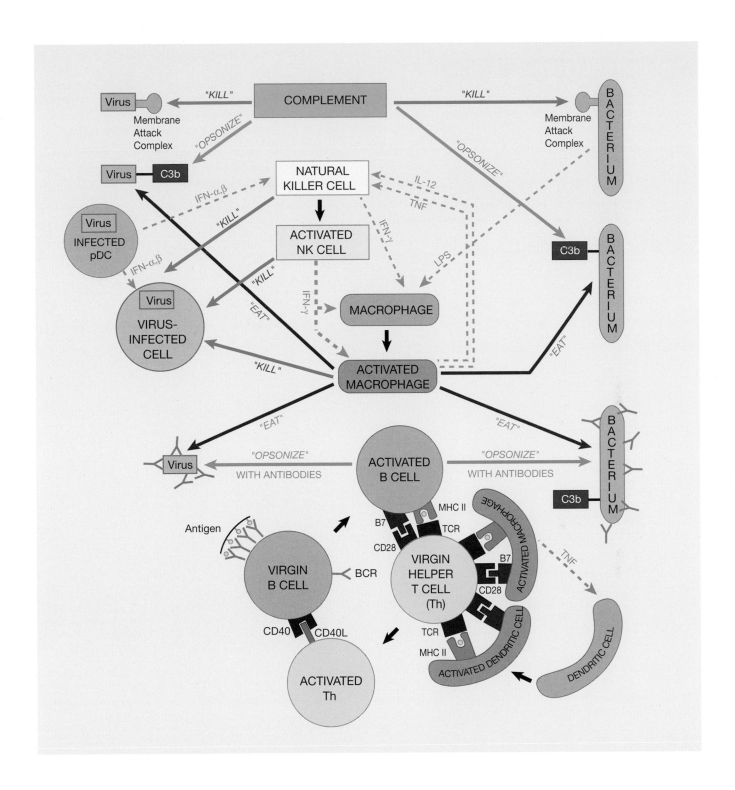

THOUGHT QUESTIONS

1. Give several reasons why antigen presentation by class I MHC molecules is important for the function of the adaptive immune system.

2. Why does antigen presentation by class II MHC molecules make good sense?

3. Describe the different roles that activated dendritic cells, activated macrophages, and activated B cells play in the presentation of antigen during the course of an infection.

4. During their lifetimes, dendritic antigen presenting cells can be "samplers," "travelers," and "presenters." Describe what DCs are doing during each of these three stages.

5. Some peptides are presented more efficiently than others. What factors influence the efficiency of presentation by class I and class II MHC molecules?

LECTURE 5   T Cell Activation

HEADS UP!

Before they can do any work, T cells must be activated. This requirement helps insure that T cells will spring into action only when there is real danger, and that only useful weapons will be mobilized. T cell activation requires recognition of the invader by the T cell's receptors, the function of co-receptor molecules that focus the attention of TCRs on the appropriate MHC molecule (class I or class II), and co-stimulation provided by an activated antigen presenting cell. There are many similarities between the ways B cells and T cells are activated – but there also are some important differences.

INTRODUCTION

The innate immune system maintains large stockpiles of weapons. This makes sense because common invaders are attacking our bodies almost continuously, and the weapons of the innate immune system are useful against a wide variety of these "everyday" enemies. In contrast, only about one in a million B or T cells will have receptors that can recognize a given invader. Consequently, it would not be wise to stockpile B or T cells, because in our entire lifetime, we probably will never encounter the invader which a particular B or T cell could defend against. Indeed, **an important feature of the adaptive immune system is that its weapons are made on demand: Only those B and T cells whose receptors can recognize the "invader *du jour*" are mobilized.** The first step in mobilizing these weapons is activation, and in this lecture, we're going to focus on how T cells are activated.

What they do once they are activated will be the subject of the next lecture.

T CELL RECEPTORS

T cell receptors (TCRs) are molecules on the surface of a T cell that function as the cell's "eyes" on the world. Without these receptors, T cells would be flying blind with no way to sense what's going on outside. T cell receptors come in two flavors: $\alpha\beta$ and $\gamma\delta$. Each type of receptor is composed of two proteins, either α and β or γ and δ. Like the heavy and light chains of the B cell receptor, the genes for α, β, γ, and δ are assembled by mixing and matching gene segments. In fact, in B and T cells, the same proteins (**RAG1** and **RAG2**) initiate the splicing of gene segments by making double-stranded breaks in chromosomal DNA. As the gene segments are mixed and matched, a "competition" ensues from which each T cell emerges with either an $\alpha\beta$ or a $\gamma\delta$ receptor, but not both. Generally, all the TCRs on a mature T cell are identical – although there are exceptions to this rule.

Traditional T cells

Over 95% of the T cells in circulation have $\alpha\beta$ **T cell receptors**, and express either **CD4** or **CD8 "co-receptor" molecules** (more about these co-receptors in a bit). The $\alpha\beta$ receptors of these "traditional" T cells recognize a complex composed of a peptide and an MHC molecule on the surface of a cell, and a "mature" T cell will have receptors that recognize peptides associated either with class I MHC molecules or with class II MHC molecules. Importantly, the $\alpha\beta$ receptors of a traditional T cell recognize both the peptide and the MHC molecule, and unlike B cells, T cells cannot undergo hypermutation to change the affinity of their TCRs for their cognate antigen.

Non-traditional T cells

In addition to traditional T cells, several kinds of "non-traditional" T cells have been discovered. T cells which have γδ **receptors** are considered to be non-traditional because, in contrast to traditional T cells, most γδ T cells do not express either the CD4 or CD8 co-receptor molecules. T cells with γδ receptors are most abundant in areas like the intestine, the uterus, and the tongue, which are in contact with the outside world. Interestingly, mice have lots of γδ T cells in the epidermal layer of their skin, but humans do not. This serves to remind us that so far as the immune system is concerned, humans are not just big mice. Human and mouse lineages diverged roughly 65 million years ago, and humans are relatively large animals that can live for a long time. In contrast, mice are small and short-lived. In fact, an "elderly" mouse is about two years old. Consequently, we would predict that, although similar, the immune systems which evolved to protect these two, very different animals would be different. And they are.

Although αβ TCRs are thought to be about as diverse as BCRs, γδ receptors are much less diverse. Moreover, the receptors of γδ T cells in the tongue and uterus tend to favor certain gene segments during rearrangement, whereas γδ receptors in the intestine prefer other combinations of gene segments. The thinking here is that, like players on the innate immune system team, γδ T cells stand watch on the "front lines," and have receptors which are "tuned" to recognize invaders that usually enter at certain locations.

There is a lot about γδ T cells which is still mysterious. For example, it is not known where these cells are educated. Traditional T cells are taught in the thymus not to react against our own self peptides, and although γδ T cells also are found in the thymus, nude mice, which lack a functional thymus, still produce functional γδ T cells. In most cases, it also is not known exactly what the receptors on γδ T cells recognize, but it is believed that, like B cells, γδ T cells focus on un-presented antigen. The receptors of some γδ T cells recognize proteins (e.g., MICA and MICB) which are expressed on the surface of cells that are under stress. Consequently, it has been postulated that γδ T cells are designed to kill cells that become stressed as the result of a microbial infection. However, the exact mission of γδ T cells is not clear.

There is another type of non-traditional T cell that is mentioned frequently, but about which relatively little is known: the **NKT cell**. In a human, only about 1% of the T cells in the blood are of this type. As its name implies, this non-traditional T cell has some of the properties of the natural killer (NK) cells of the innate system, and some of the properties of traditional T cells of the adaptive immune system. NKT cells mature in the thymus and have αβ receptors. However, in contrast to the αβ receptors of traditional T cells, which are incredibly diverse, the repertoire of receptors expressed by NKT cells is quite limited. In addition, the receptors of NKT cells recognize lipids presented by non-classical, CD1 MHC molecules instead of protein fragments presented by class I or class II MHC molecules. It has been proposed that NKT cells evolved as a weapon designed to protect us against microbes like tuberculosis which produce characteristic lipid molecules. However, normal mice and mice that have been engineered to lack NKT cells are equally susceptible to infection with TB, and, so far, it is not clear how important NKT cells are in protecting humans against bacterial infections.

Because much more is known about traditional T cells than about their non-traditional cousins, and because traditional T cells seem to be the ones that are most important for protecting us from disease, we will limit our discussion in this book to T cells of the traditional variety.

HOW A T CELL'S RECEPTORS SIGNAL

Once a TCR has recognized its cognate antigen presented by an MHC molecule, the next step is to transmit a signal from the surface of the T cell, where recognition takes place, to the nucleus of the T cell. The idea is that for the T cell to switch from a resting state to a state of activation, gene expression must be altered, and these genes are, of course, located in the cell's nucleus. Normally, this type of signaling across the cell membrane involves a transmembrane protein that has two parts: an external region which binds to a molecule (called a ligand) that is outside the cell, plus an internal region that initiates a biochemical cascade which conveys the "ligand bound" signal to the nucleus. Here the TCR runs into a bit of a problem. As is true of the BCR, the αβ TCR has a perfectly fine extracellular domain that can bind to its ligand (the combination of MHC molecule and peptide), but the cytoplasmic tails of the α and β proteins are only about three amino acids long – way too short to signal.

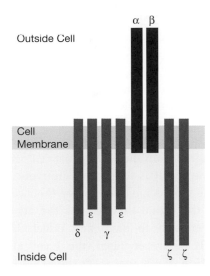

Outside Cell

α   β

Cell Membrane

δ   γ   ε   ε   ζ   ζ

Inside Cell

To handle the signaling chores, Mother Nature had to add a few bells and whistles to the TCR: a complex of proteins collectively called **CD3**. In humans, this signaling complex is made up of four different proteins: γ, δ, ε, and ζ (gamma, delta, epsilon, and zeta). The CD3 proteins are anchored in the cell membrane, and have cytoplasmic tails that are long enough to signal just fine. Please note, however, that the γ and δ proteins that are part of the CD3 complex are not the same as the γ and δ proteins that make up the γδ T cell receptor.

The whole complex of proteins (α, β, γ, δ, ε, ζ) is transported to the cell surface as a unit. If any one of these proteins fails to be made, you don't get a TCR on the surface. Consequently, most immunologists consider the functional, mature TCR to be this whole complex of proteins. After all, the α and β proteins are great for recognition, but they can't signal. And together, the γ, δ, ε, and ζ proteins signal just fine, but they are totally blind to what's going on outside the cell. You need both parts to make it work. As with BCRs, **signaling involves clustering TCRs together in one area of the T cell surface.** When this happens, a threshold number of kinase enzymes are recruited by the cytoplasmic tails of the CD3 proteins, and the activation signal is dispatched to the nucleus.

When the α and β chains of the TCR were first discovered, it was thought that the TCR was just an on/off switch whose only function was to signal activation. But now that you have heard about the CD3 proteins, let me ask you: Does this look like a simple on/off switch? No way! Mother Nature certainly wouldn't make an on/off switch with six proteins. No, **this TCR is quite**

versatile. It can send signals that result in very different outcomes, depending on how, when, and where it is triggered. For example, in the thymus, if a T cell's receptors recognize MHC plus self peptide, the TCRs trigger the T cell to commit suicide to prevent autoimmunity. Later in its life, if its TCRs recognize their cognate antigen presented by MHC molecules, but that T cell does not receive the required co-stimulatory signals, the T cell may be neutered (anergized) so it can't function. And, of course, when a TCR is presented with its cognate antigen, and co-stimulatory signals are available, the TCR can signal activation. So this same T cell receptor, depending on the situation, signals death, anergy, or activation. In fact, there are now documented cases in which the alteration of a single amino acid in a presented peptide can change the signal from activation to death! Clearly this is no on/off switch, and immunologists are working very hard to understand exactly how TCR signaling is "wired," and what factors influence the signaling outcomes.

CD4 AND CD8 CO-RECEPTORS

In addition to the T cell receptor, there are two more molecules which are involved in antigen recognition by T cells – the **CD4 and CD8 co-receptors**. Now, doesn't it seem that Mother Nature got carried away when she added on these CD4 and CD8 co-receptors? I mean, there are already two proteins, α and β, to use for antigen recognition, and four more, γ, δ, ε, and ζ, to use for signaling. Wouldn't you think that would do it? Apparently not, so there must be essential features of the system that require CD4 and CD8 co-receptors. Let's see what these might be.

Killer T cells and helper T cells perform two very different functions, and they "look at" two different molecules, class I or class II MHC, respectively, to get their cues. But how do CTLs know to focus on peptides presented by class I molecules – and how do Th cells know to scan APCs for peptides presented by class II? After all, it wouldn't be so great if a CTL got confused, recognized a class II–peptide complex on an APC, and killed that antigen presenting cell. So here's where CD4 and CD8 come in. **CTLs generally express CD8, and Th cells usually express CD4. These co-receptor molecules are designed to clip onto either class I MHC (CD8) or class II MHC molecules (CD4).**

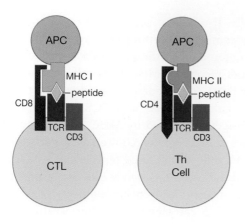

These "clips" strengthen the adhesion between the T cell and the APC somewhat, so **CD4 and CD8 co-receptors help focus the attention of Th cells and CTLs on the proper MHC molecule.** But there is more to the story. It turns out that CD4 and CD8 are signaling molecules just like the CD3 complex of proteins. Both CD4 and CD8 have tails that extend through the cell's plasma membrane and into the cytoplasm, and both of these tails have the right characteristics to signal. In contrast to CD3 molecules, which are glued rather tightly to the αβ T cell receptor on the cell surface, the CD4 and CD8 co-receptors usually are only loosely associated with the TCR/CD3 proteins. The idea is that **after a TCR has engaged its cognate antigen presented by an MHC molecule, the CD4 or CD8 co-receptors then clip on, help stabilize the TCR–MHC–peptide interaction, and strengthen the signal sent by the TCR.**

When T cells begin maturing in the thymus, they express both types of co-receptors on their surface. Immunologists call them CD4$^+$CD8$^+$ or "double-positive" cells. Then, as they mature, expression of one or the other of these co-receptors is downregulated, and a cell becomes either CD4$^+$ or CD8$^+$. So how does a given T cell decide whether it will express the CD4 or the CD8 co-receptor when it grows up? Although there is still some disagreement about this process, the latest thinking is that the type of MHC molecule the TCR recognizes determines this choice. If a T cell's receptors have the right structure to recognize a class I MHC molecule, that T cell downregulates expression of CD4, and only displays the CD8 co-receptor molecule on its surface. On the other hand, if a T cell's receptors prefer to bind to a class II MHC molecule, that T cell is "instructed" to continue to express the CD4 but not the CD8 co-receptor.

CO-STIMULATION

In naive T cells, the "connection" between the T cell's receptors and the cell's nucleus is not very good. It's as if the T cell had an electrical system in which a large resistor were placed between the sensor (the TCR) and the piece of equipment it is designed to regulate (gene expression in the nucleus). Because of this "resistor," a lot of the signal from the TCR is lost as it travels to the nucleus. The result is that a prohibitively large number of TCRs would have to engage their cognate antigen before the signal that reaches the nucleus would be strong enough to have any effect. If, however, while the TCRs are engaged, the T cell also receives **co-stimulation**, the signal from the TCRs is amplified many times, so that fewer (probably about 100-fold fewer) TCRs must be engaged to activate a naive T cell. Although a number of different molecules have been identified which can co-stimulate T cells, certainly the best studied examples are the B7 proteins (B7-1 and B7-2) which are expressed on the surface of antigen presenting cells. B7 molecules provide co-stimulation to T cells by plugging into receptor molecules called CD28 on the T cell's surface.

So in addition to having their T cell receptors ligated by MHC–peptide, naive T cells also must receive co-stimulatory signals before they can be activated. Co-stimulation can be thought of as an "amplifier" that strengthens the "I'm engaged" signal sent by a T cell's receptors, thereby lowering the threshold number of TCRs which must be crosslinked by MHC–peptide complexes. Interestingly, once a naive T cell has been activated, the connection between the TCRs and the nucleus strengthens. It is as if an experienced T cell has been "re-wired" so that the resistor present in a naive T cell is bypassed. As a result of this re-wiring, in an experienced T cell, amplification of the TCR signal is not as important as it is in a virgin T cell. Consequently, **experienced T cells have a reduced requirement for co-stimulation.**

A TIME-LAPSE PHOTO OF HELPER T CELL ACTIVATION

In the lymph nodes, helper T cells quickly scan dendritic cells to see if their cognate antigen is being displayed. A single dendritic cell typically hosts about 1000 such "visits" each hour. If a T cell does find a dendritic cell displaying its cognate antigen, the T cell "lingers," because complete activation of a naive helper T cell usually takes several hours. During this time, a number of important events take place. First, adhesion molecules on the surface of the dendritic cell bind to their adhesion partners on the T cell, helping keep the two cells together. Next, the CD4 co-receptor molecules on the surface of the T cell clip onto the class II MHC molecules on the dendritic cell and strengthen the interaction between the two cells. In addition, the engagement of its TCRs upregulates the expression of adhesion molecules on the Th cell surface, strengthening the "glue" that holds the APC and the T cell together. This is important, because **the initial binding between a TCR and an MHC–peptide complex is actually rather weak to allow for rapid scanning. Consequently, the Velcro-like adhesion molecules are extremely important for T cell activation.** The clustering of TCRs and adhesion molecules at the point of contact between an APC and a T cell results in the formation of what immunologists call an **immunological synapse**.

Engagement of a helper T cell's receptors also upregulates expression of CD40L proteins on its surface, and when these proteins plug into the CD40 proteins on the surface of a dendritic cell, several remarkable things happen. Although mature dendritic cells express MHC and co-stimulatory molecules (e.g., B7) when they first enter lymph nodes, the expression level of these proteins increases when CD40 proteins on the APC are engaged by the CD40L proteins on a Th cell. In addition, engagement of a dendritic cell's CD40 proteins prolongs the life of the dendritic cell. This extension of a "useful" dendritic cell's life span makes perfect sense. It insures that the particular dendritic cells which are presenting a T cell's cognate antigen will stick around long enough to help activate a lot of these T cells. So **the interaction between a dendritic cell and a naive helper T cell is not just one-way. These cells actually perform an activation "dance" in which they stimulate each other. The end result of this cooperation is that the dendritic cell becomes a more potent antigen presenting cell, and the Th cell is activated to express the high levels of CD40L required for helping activate B cells.**

After activation is complete, the helper T cell and the antigen presenting cell part. The APC then goes on to activate other T cells, while the recently activated Th cells proliferate to build up their numbers. During an infection, a single activated T cell can give rise to about 10 000 daughter cells during the first week or so of proliferation. This proliferation is driven by growth factors such as IL-2. Naive T cells can make some IL-2, but they don't have IL-2 receptors on their surface – so they can't respond to this cytokine. In contrast, activated Th cells produce large amounts of IL-2, and they also express receptors for this cytokine on their surface. As a result, newly activated helper T cells stimulate their own proliferation. **This coupling of activation to the upregulation of growth factor receptors is the essence of clonal selection: Those Th cells which are selected for activation (because their TCRs recognize an invader) upregulate their growth factor receptors, and proliferate to form a clone.**

So the sequence of events during the activation of a helper T cell is this: Adhesion molecules mediate weak binding between the Th and the APC while TCRs engage their cognate antigen presented by the APC. Receptor engagement strengthens the adhesion between the two cells, and upregulates CD40L expression on the Th cell. CD40L then binds to CD40 on the APC and stimulates expression of MHC and co-stimulatory molecules on the APC surface. The co-stimulation provided by the APC amplifies the "TCR engaged" signal, making activation of the Th cell more efficient. When activation is complete, the cells disengage, and the Th cell proliferates, driven by growth factors which bind to receptors that appear on the Th cell surface as a result of activation. This proliferation produces a clone of helper T cells which can recognize the invader advertised by the antigen presenting cell.

HOW KILLER T CELLS ARE ACTIVATED

For a helper T cell to be activated, its receptors must recognize their cognate antigen displayed by class II MHC molecules on the surface of an activated dendritic cell, and the Th cell must also receive co-stimulatory signals from that same dendritic cell. This requirement that two cells (the Th cell and the DC) agree that there has been an invasion is a powerful safeguard against the activation of "rogue" helper T cells – cells which might direct an attack against our own tissues, causing autoimmune disease.

Although the events involved in the activation of helper T cells are pretty clear, the picture of how naive killer T cells are activated is still rather fuzzy. Until recently, it was believed that for a naive killer T cell to be activated, three cells needed to be involved: a CTL with receptors that recognized the invader; an activated dendritic cell, which was using its class I MHC molecules to present fragments of the invader's proteins to the CTL; and an activated helper T cell which was providing "help" to the CTL. One way this might happen would be for the dendritic cell, the Th cell, and the CTL to engage in a *ménage à trois*. There is, however, a potential problem with this scenario. Early in an infection, there are very few of any of these cells around. Consequently, the probability is quite small that a helper T cell and a killer T cell would simultaneously find a dendritic cell which is presenting their cognate antigens.

Experiments have now shown that, in response to an invasion by microbes which can infect cells (the microbes that CTLs are designed to defend against), T cell help is not required during the initial activation of killer T cells. A two-cell interaction between a naive CTL and an activated dendritic cell is sufficient. During this meeting, the CTL's receptors recognize their cognate antigen displayed by class I MHC molecules on the dendritic cell, and they receive the co-stimulation they need from that same dendritic cell. What this means is that a naive killer T cell can be activated in a way that is analogous to the way a naive Th cell is activated: by encountering an activated dendritic cell.

Requiring only a two-cell interaction for the activation of naive Th cells and CTLs makes perfect sense in terms of getting the adaptive immune system fired up before invaders take over completely. However, activation of naive killer T cells without Th cell help does raise an important question: If Th cells are supposed to be orchestrating the immune response, just what is their contribution in terms of giving directions to killer T cells?

Although a single CTL is capable of killing many target cells sequentially, thousands of cells usually are infected during an attack. Consequently, many CTLs are required to repulse a serious attack. Killer T cells require IL-2 for continued proliferation, and activated helper T cells are the major supplier of this growth factor. If there is a dangerous invasion, many Th cells will be activated. These cells will produce a lot of IL-2, which will encourage massive proliferation of activated CTLs. So by supplying a killer T cell's favorite growth factor, IL-2, Th cells can help control the strength of the CTL response.

Experiments also have shown that when CTLs are activated without Th cell help, they do proliferate somewhat to build up their numbers and they can kill infected cells. Nevertheless, these "helpless" CTLs do not kill with high efficiency, and they do not live very long. It is as if helpless activation of CTLs results in a small "burst" of killer T cells designed to deal quickly with invaders early in an infection. In contrast, in order to efficiently activate long-lived killer T cells or to generate memory killer T cells (cells which can defend against a subsequent invasion by the same attacker) assistance from helper T cells is required. And this, of course, brings us back to the question of how CTLs can be fully activated by Th cells and DCs without requiring a three-cell interaction.

One possibility, the "sequential model," postulates that when helper T cells are activated, the dendritic cells which activate them become "licensed" to activate CTLs – thus avoiding the need for all three cells to meet simultaneously. It has also been demonstrated that when an activated dendritic cell and a helper T cell "hook up," chemokines are generated which can attract naive killer T cells to their location, making a *ménage à trois* more likely. Moreover, the probability of such a three-cell interaction also is increased by the fact that the meeting between an activated dendritic cell and a helper T cell typically lasts for several hours. Consequently, cytokine-directed migration and extended Th–APC interaction times could give that rare CTL which also recognizes the invader a better chance to join the party. Finally, relatively late in an immune response, there will be many activated dendritic cells, Th cells, and killer T cells present in lymph nodes and other secondary lymphoid organs – perhaps enough of each of these cell types to make a three-cell interaction probable. My guess is that killer T cells can be activated by several of these mechanisms. But stay tuned!

FAIL-SAFE ACTIVATION

For either a naive helper T cell or a virgin CTL to be activated, the T cell must first recognize its cognate antigen presented by an antigen presenting cell. This is true even for helper T cell-independent activation of CTLs. As a consequence of this requirement for antigen presentation during activation, a fail-safe system is set up in which the decision to activate a T cell always involves more than one cell. This helps insure that the powerful weapons of the adaptive immune system only come into play when there is a genuine threat, and makes it less likely that a T cell will turn its weapons inward on its host.

REVIEW

There are many similarities between the ways B cells and T cells are activated. BCRs and TCRs both have "recognition" proteins that extend outside the cell, and which are incredibly diverse because they are made by mixing and matching gene segments. For the BCR, these recognition proteins are the light and heavy chains that make up the antibody molecule. For the TCR, the molecules that recognize antigen are the α and β proteins. TCRs and BCRs have cytoplasmic tails that are too short to signal recognition, so additional molecules are required for this purpose. For the BCR, these signaling proteins are called Igα and Igβ. For the TCR, signaling involves a complex of proteins called CD3.

For B and T cells to be activated, their receptors must be clustered by antigen, because this crosslinking brings together many of their signaling molecules in a small region of the cell. When the density of signaling molecules is great enough, an enzymatic chain reaction is set off that conveys the "receptor engaged" signal to the cell's nucleus. There, in the "brain center" of the cell, genes involved in activation are turned off or on as a result of this signal.

Although crosslinking of receptors is essential for the activation of B and T cells, it is not enough. Naive B and T cells also require co-stimulatory signals that are not antigen specific. This two-signal requirement for activation sets up a fail-safe system which protects against the inappropriate activation of B and T cells. For B cell activation, a helper T cell can provide co-stimulation through surface proteins called CD40L that plug into CD40 proteins on the B cell surface. B cells also can be co-stimulated by "danger signals," including invader-specific molecular signatures or battle cytokines. For T cells, co-stimulation usually involves B7 proteins on an activated dendritic cell that engage CD28 proteins on the surface of the T cell.

Both BCRs and TCRs can associate with co-receptor molecules which serve to amplify the signal that the BCRs and TCRs send. For B cells, this co-receptor recognizes antigen that has been opsonized by complement. If the BCR recognizes an antigen, and if that antigen also is "decorated" with complement protein fragments, the antigen serves as a "clamp" that brings the BCR and the complement receptor together on the surface of the B cell, greatly amplifying the "receptor engaged" signal. As a consequence, B cells are much more easily activated (many fewer BCRs need to be crosslinked) by antigen that has been opsonized by complement.

T cells also have co-receptors. Th cells express CD4 co-receptor molecules on their surface, and CTLs express CD8 co-receptors. When a TCR binds to antigen presented by an MHC molecule, the co-receptor on the T cell surface clips onto the MHC molecule. This serves to strengthen the signal that is sent by the TCR to the nucleus, so that the T cell is more easily activated (fewer TCRs need to be crosslinked). These co-receptors only work with the "right" MHC types: class I for CTLs with CD8 co-receptors, and class II for Th cells with CD4 co-receptors. Consequently, co-receptors really are "focus" molecules. The B cell co-receptor helps B cells focus on antigens that have already been identified by the complement system as dangerous (those that have been opsonized). The CD4 co-receptor focuses the attention of Th cells on antigens displayed by class II MHC molecules, and the CD8 co-receptor focuses CTLs on antigens displayed by class I MHC molecules.

Of course, there is an important difference between what B cells and T cells "look at." The BCR recognizes antigen in its "natural" state – that is, antigen which has not been chopped up and bound to MHC molecules. This antigen can be a protein or almost any other organic molecule (e.g., a carbohydrate or a fat). In contrast, the $\alpha\beta$ receptors of traditional T cells only recognize fragments of proteins presented by MHC molecules. And whereas a B cell's receptors only bind to one thing – its cognate antigen – the TCR binds to both the presented peptide and the MHC molecule. Because the universe of antigens recognized by the BCR includes proteins, carbohydrates, and fats, B cells can respond to a greater variety of invaders than can T cells. On the other hand, because the TCR looks at small fragments of proteins, it can recognize targets that are hidden from view of the BCR in an intact and tightly folded protein.

Another difference between B cells and T cells is that during an infection, the BCR can undergo somatic hypermutation and selection. So B cells can "draw from the deck" to try to get a better hand. In contrast, the TCR does not hypermutate, so T cells must be satisfied with the cards they are dealt.

THOUGHT QUESTIONS

1. What is the difference between a co-receptor and co-stimulation? Give examples and tell why each is important for B or T cell activation.

2. Why are cellular adhesion molecules important during T cell activation? Don't these "sticky" molecules just slow the process down?

3. What happens when dendritic cells and helper T cells "dance"?

4. Essentially all players on the innate and adaptive immune system teams must be activated before they can "get into the game." Trace the steps in the "activation cascade" which begins when an LPS-carrying, Gram-negative bacterium enters a wound, and which ends when antibodies are produced that can recognize the bacterium.

5. Mother Nature uses "fail-safe technology" to prevent inappropriate activation of the immune system. Can you give several examples?

T Cells at Work

INTRODUCTION

Once helper T cells and killer T cells have been activated, they are ready to go to work – to become what immunologists call **effector cells**. The primary job of an effector CTL is to kill cells that have been infected by viruses or bacteria. Effector helper T cells have two main duties. First, they can remain in the blood and lymphatic circulation and travel from node to node, providing help for B cells or for killer T cells. In addition, effector helper T cells can exit blood vessels at the sites where a battle is going on to provide help for the soldiers of the innate and adaptive immune systems.

HELPER T CELLS AS CYTOKINE FACTORIES

Helper T cells can produce many different cytokines – protein molecules which they use to communicate with the rest of the immune system. As the "quarterback" of the immune system team, the helper T cell uses cytokines to "call the plays." These include cytokines such as TNF, IFN-γ, IL-4, IL-5, IL-6, IL-10, IL-17, and IL-21. However, a single Th cell doesn't secrete all these different cytokines. In fact, Th cells tend to secrete subsets of cytokines – subsets which are appropriate to orchestrate an immune defense against particular invaders. So far, three major subsets have been identified: **Th1**, **Th2**, and **Th17**. You shouldn't take this to mean, however, that there are only three different combinations of cytokines that can be secreted by Th cells. In fact, immunologists initially had a hard time finding helper T cells that secreted exactly the Th1 or Th2 cytokine subsets in humans. Clearly, there are helper T cells which give off mixtures of cytokines that don't conform to the Th1/Th2/Th17 paradigm. Nevertheless, this concept turns out to be quite useful in trying to make sense of the combination of cytokines (the cytokine "profile") that Th cells produce. I also should mention that in addition to these three Th subsets which are involved in activating the immune system, there is a subset of Th cells which functions to suppress the immune response. We will discuss those "Treg" cells in subsequent lectures.

Of course, all of this begs the question: How does a helper T cell know which cytokines are appropriate for a given situation? Well, as any football fan knows, behind every good quarterback, there is a good coach.

THE DENDRITIC CELL AS "COACH" OF THE IMMUNE SYSTEM TEAM

For a helper T cell to make an informed decision about which cytokines to make, at least two pieces of information are required. First, it's necessary to know what type of invader the immune system is dealing with. Is it a virus, a bacterium, a parasite, or a fungus? Second, it is essential to determine where in the body the invaders are located. Are they in the respiratory tract, the digestive tract, or the big toe? Virgin helper T cells don't have direct access to either type of information. After all, they are busy circulating through the blood and lymph, trying to find their cognate antigen. What is needed is an "observer" who actually has been at the battle site, who has collected the pertinent information, and who can pass it along to the helper T cell. And which of the immune system cells could qualify as such an observer? The dendritic antigen presenting cell, of course!

Just as a football coach scouts the opposing team and formulates a game plan, so a dendritic cell, acting as the "coach" of the immune system team, collects information on the invasion, and decides how the immune system should react. That's why dendritic cells are so important. They don't just turn naive helper T cells and killer T cells on. **Dendritic cells actually function as the "brains" of the immune system, processing the information pertaining to the invasion, and producing a plan of action.**

What are the inputs that dendritic cells integrate to produce the game plan? These are of two types. The first input comes to the dendritic cell through the pattern-recognition receptors we discussed in Lecture 2. These cellular receptors recognize conserved patterns that are characteristic of various classes of invaders. For example, Toll-like receptor 4 (TLR4) senses the presence of LPS, which is a molecule that is a component of the outer cell membrane of Gram-negative bacteria. TLR4 also can detect proteins made by certain viruses. TLR2 specializes in identifying proteins that are "signatures" of Gram-positive bacteria. TLR3 recognizes the double-stranded RNA produced during many viral infections. And TLR9 recognizes the unmethylated DNA dinucleotide, CpG, which is characteristic of bacterial DNA.

Although TLRs were the first pattern-recognition receptors to be characterized, additional families of pattern-recognition receptors have now been discovered. Consequently, the emerging picture is that different types of antigen presenting cells (e.g., dendritic cells or macrophages) in different parts of the body display distinct sets of these pattern-recognition receptors which are "tuned" to recognize various structural features of common microbial invaders. By integrating the signals from these diverse pattern-recognition receptors, an APC gathers information on the type of invader to be defended against.

The second "scouting report" dendritic cells employ when formulating their game plan is received through various cytokine receptors on their surface. Because different pathogens elicit the production of different cytokines during an infection, dendritic cells can learn a lot about an invader by sensing the cytokine environment. So **dendritic cells out on the front lines collect "intelligence" about an invader through pattern-recognition receptors and cytokine receptors. It is then up to the dendritic cell to "decode" these inputs in order to discern the type of invasion, and to decide which weapons need to be mobilized.**

Cells in different areas of the body (e.g., skin cells or cells that underlie the intestines) produce characteristic mixtures of cytokines in response to invaders, and these cytokines provide dendritic cells with information about the area of the body that is under attack. In fact, these cytokines imprint dendritic cells with a "regional identity." And this ability to **remember their "roots" helps DCs dispatch the weapons of the adaptive immune system to the parts of the body where they are needed.**

But how is the dendritic cell's game plan conveyed to the Th cell – the cell that will direct the action? There are two ways that the coach instructs the quarterback. First, the mixture of co-stimulatory molecules displayed on the surface of an activated dendritic cell will depend on the type of invader the DC has encountered. These co-stimulatory molecules can "plug into" receptor molecules on the surface of helper T cells to pass this information along. Although B7 is the best-studied co-stimulatory molecule, other co-stimulatory molecules have been identified, and more are certain to be discovered.

In addition to co-stimulatory surface molecules, activated dendritic cells produce cytokines which also can convey information to the helper T cell. So the bottom line is this: **Co-stimulatory molecules and cytokines are used by dendritic cells to pass along the "game plan" to helper T cells. And the particular combination of co-stimulatory molecules and cytokines which a dendritic cell offers to a Th cell will depend on what the dendritic cell has observed at the battle scene.** To get a better idea of how this all works, let's look more closely at the Th1, Th2, and Th17 subsets of cytokines.

Th1 HELPER T CELLS

If you have a puncture wound that results in a bacterial infection or if you are attacked by a virus that replicates in the tissues, resident dendritic cells will be alerted through their pattern-recognition receptors and by receiving battle cytokines produced by macrophages and other cells in the inflamed tissues. These signals activate the dendritic cell and imprint it with the special characteristics of an APC which has observed a bacterial or viral infection in the tissues. The details of exactly how this is accomplished aren't clear yet, but the result is that when this DC leaves such a battle site and travels through the lymph to a nearby lymph node, it will produce the cytokine IL-12. And when the IL-12-producing DC presents the battle antigens it has acquired to a virgin helper T cell, that Th cell will be instructed to become a helper T cell which produces the "classical" Th1 cytokines: TNF, IFN-γ, and IL-2.

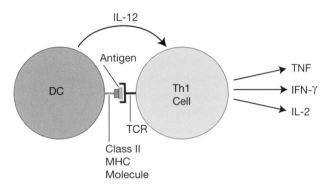

Why these particular cytokines? Let's see what these cytokines do. The TNF secreted by Th1 helper T cells helps activate macrophages and natural killer cells. However, macrophages only stay activated for a limited time. They are lazy fellows which like to go back to resting and garbage collecting. Fortunately, the IFN-γ produced by Th1 cells acts as a "prod" that keeps macrophages fired up and engaged in the battle. IFN-γ also influences B cells during class switching to produce human IgG3 antibodies. These antibodies are especially good at opsonizing viruses and bacteria and at fixing complement.

NK cells can kill three or four target cells in about 16 hours, but then they "tire out." The IL-2 produced by Th1 cells can "recharge" NK cells, enabling them to kill some more. In addition, IL-2 is a growth factor which stimulates the proliferation of CTLs, NK cells, and Th1 cells themselves – so that more of these important weapons will be available to deal with the attack.

Altogether, **the Th1 cytokines are the perfect package to help defend against a viral or bacterial attack in the tissues. The Th1 cytokines instruct the innate and adaptive systems to mobilize cells and produce antibodies that are especially effective against these invaders, and these cytokines also keep the warriors of the immune system fired up until the invaders have been defeated.**

Th2 HELPER T CELLS

Now suppose that you have been infected by a parasite (e.g., hook worms) or you have eaten some food that is contaminated with pathogenic bacteria. In the tissues that line your intestines, a battle will be raging. Dendritic cells from that area will travel to nearby lymph nodes, and will activate those helper T cells which have T cell receptors that can recognize the worm or bacterial antigens presented by the DC. This interaction results in helper T cells which are "programmed" to produce the Th2 subset of cytokines, which includes IL-4, IL-5, and IL-13.

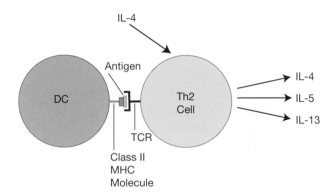

Why IL-4, IL-5, and IL-13, you ask? IL-4 is a growth factor that stimulates the proliferation of helper T cells which have committed to secrete the Th2 profile of cytokines. So, like Th1 cells, Th2 cells produce their own growth factor. IL-4 also is a growth factor for B cells, and this cytokine can influence B cells to class switch to produce IgE antibodies – powerful weapons against parasites such as hook worms. IL-5 is a cytokine which encourages B cells to produce IgA antibodies, antibodies that are especially useful against bacteria which invade via the digestive tract. And IL-13 stimulates the production of mucus in the intestines. This helps prevent more intestinal parasites or pathogenic bacteria from breaching the intestinal barrier and entering the tissues. So **the Th2 cytokine profile is just the ticket if you need to defend against parasites or pathogenic bacteria that have invaded via the digestive tract.**

In the figure above, you will notice that IL-4, which causes a naive Th cell to commit to becoming a Th2 cell, does not come from the dendritic cell. Of course, once the helper T cell commits to the Th2 cytokine profile, there will be plenty of IL-4 around – because this is one of the cytokines Th2 cells secrete. However, the initial source of IL-4 required for Th2 commitment has not yet been identified.

Th17 HELPER T CELLS

The existence of helper T cells which produce the Th17 cytokine profile is a recent discovery, and less is known about Th17 cells than about Th1 and Th2 helper T cells. One reason for this is that Th17 cells function, at least in part, in the defense against fungi – and the immune system's response to a fungal attack is not nearly so well researched as the immune defense against bacteria or viruses. Consequently, the story on Th17 cells is still incomplete, but here's the emerging picture.

If a dendritic cell is stationed in an area of the body which is being attacked by fungi (e.g., a vaginal yeast infection) or by certain extracellular bacteria, that DC will travel to a nearby lymph node to activate helper T cells which recognize the antigens the DC is presenting. These traveling dendritic cells will produce TGFβ and IL-6, which together with co-stimulatory molecules, influence newly activated helper T cells to produce the Th17 subset of cytokines, which includes IL-17 and IL-21.

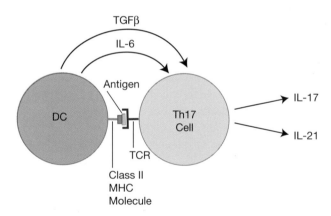

IL-21 encourages uncommitted Th cells to become Th17 cells, and this increases the number of Th17 cells available to battle the fungus. Secretion of the "signature cytokine," IL-17, results in the recruitment of massive numbers of neutrophils to the site of infection. These neutrophils help defend against pathogens against which Th1 and Th2 cells are relatively ineffective, including fungi and some extracellular bacteria – bacteria which do not enter cells. Indeed, patients who have a genetic defect in IL-17 secretion suffer from devastating fungal infections (e.g., infection with the common yeast, *Candida albicans*) even though their Th1 and Th2 helper T cells function normally. IL-17 and IL-21 influence B cells to produce antibody classes that can opsonize fungi or bacteria and can activate the complement system. So if you are attacked by fungi or extracellular bacteria, the cytokines secreted by Th17 cells are there to help protect you.

Th0 HELPER T CELLS

Some helper T cells (the **Th0** cells) remain "unbiased" when they first are activated, retaining the ability to produce a wide range of cytokines. It appears that DCs tell these helper T cells where to go, but not what to do. However, once Th0 cells reach the battle scene, the cytokine environment they encounter there causes them to commit to the cytokine profile required for the defense. For example, when Th0 cells exit the blood to fight a bacterial infection in the tissues, they encounter an environment rich in IL-12. This is because Th1 cells that are already fighting bacteria there produce IFN-γ. This cytokine, together with danger signals like the bacterial molecule LPS, activates tissue macrophages, which secrete large amounts of IL-12. And when Th0 cells receive the IL-12 signal, they "realize" what type of battle is being fought, and commit to becoming Th1 cells – which produce the cytokines needed to defend against bacteria.

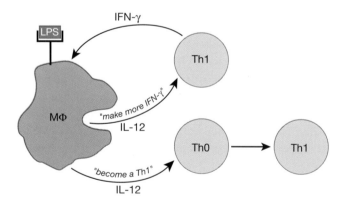

Likewise, Th0 cells can become Th2 or Th17 cells when they reach a battle site that is rich in IL-4 or IL-6 and TGFβ, respectively. So previously uncommitted Th0 cells can be "converted" by the cytokine environment at the scene of the battle to become Th1, Th2, or Th17 cells.

LOCKING IN THE HELPER T CELL PROFILE

Once helper T cells commit to a particular cytokine profile, they begin to secrete cytokines which encourage the proliferation of that particular type of Th cell – be it Th1,

Th2, or Th17. This sets up a positive feedback loop which results in even more of the "selected" Th cells being produced.

In addition to positive feedback, there is also negative feedback at work. For example, IFN-γ made by Th1 cells actually decreases the rate of proliferation of Th2 cells, so that fewer Th2 cells will be produced. And one of the Th2 cytokines, IL-10, acts to decrease the rate of proliferation of Th1 cells. **The result of all this positive and negative feedback is a large number of helper T cells which are strongly biased toward the production of a certain subset of cytokines.**

There is an important point about helper T cell bias which I want to be sure you understand. **Cytokines have a very limited range.** They can travel only short distances in the body before they are captured by cellular receptors or are degraded. Consequently, **when we talk about helper T cells being biased toward secreting a certain cytokine profile, we are talking about something very local.** Clearly, you wouldn't want every Th cell in your body to be of the Th1 type, because then you'd have no way to defend against a respiratory infection. Conversely, you wouldn't want to have only Th2 cells, because the IgA or IgE antibodies made in response to the Th2 cytokines would be useless if you get a bacterial infection in your big toe. In fact, **it is the local nature of cytokine signaling which gives the immune system the flexibility to simultaneously mount defenses against many different invaders that threaten different parts of the body.**

It is also important to note that dendritic cells are members of the innate system team. Consequently, **the innate immune system not only informs the adaptive system when there is danger, it also "coaches" the adaptive system to insure that the appropriate weapons are sent to the right places.**

DELAYED-TYPE HYPERSENSITIVITY

There is an example of "signal calling" by Th cells that I think you'll find interesting. It is termed **delayed-type hypersensitivity (DTH)**, and it was first observed by Robert Koch when he was studying tuberculosis back in the latter part of the nineteenth century. Koch purified a protein, tuberculin, from the bacterium which causes tuberculosis, and used this protein to devise his famous "tuberculin skin test." If you've had this test, you'll recall that a nurse injected something under your skin,

and told you to check that area in a few days. If the spot where you were injected became red and swollen, you were instructed to come back in to see the doctor. Here's what that's all about.

The "something" you were injected with was Koch's tuberculin protein. If you have active TB or have been infected with it in the past, your immune system will include memory, Th1-type helper T cells that were made in response to the infection. When the nurse injects the tuberculin protein, dendritic cells stationed beneath the skin take up the protein and present tuberculin peptides to these memory cells – and they are reactivated. Now the fun begins, because these Th cells secrete IFN-γ and TNF – Th1-type cytokines that activate resident tissue macrophages near the site of injection, and help recruit neutrophils and additional macrophages to the area. The result is a local inflammatory reaction with redness and swelling: the signal that your TB test is positive. Of course, the reason you have to wait several days for the test to "develop" is that memory helper T cells must be reactivated, proliferate, and produce those all-important cytokines that orchestrate the inflammatory reaction.

On the other hand, if you have never been exposed to the tuberculosis bacterium, you will have no memory helper T cells to reactivate. Without the cytokines supplied by activated Th cells, there will be no inflammatory reaction to the tuberculin protein, and your skin test will be scored as negative.

What is interesting here is that **delayed-type hypersensitivity is both specific and non-specific. The specificity comes from Th cells that direct the immune response after recognizing the tuberculin peptide presented by dendritic cells. The non-specific part of the reaction involves the neutrophils and macrophages that are recruited and activated by cytokines secreted by the Th cells.** This is yet another example of the cooperation that goes on between the adaptive and innate immune systems.

You may be wondering why the tuberculin used for the test doesn't activate naive T cells, so that the next time you are tested, you will get a positive reaction. The reason is that the tuberculin protein does not, by itself, cause an inflammatory reaction (i.e., a battle situation), and you remember that dendritic cells only mature and carry antigen to a lymph node if a battle is on. Consequently, if a protein that is injected under your skin is judged by the innate system not to be dangerous, the adaptive immune system will not be activated. This illustrates again how important the innate immune system is for initiating an immune response: **If your innate system does not recognize an invader as dangerous and put up a fight, your adaptive system usually will just ignore the intrusion.**

HOW CTLs KILL

So far in this lecture, we have discussed what activated helper T cells do. Now it is time to focus on killer T cells. Once a CTL has been activated, it proliferates rapidly to build up its numbers. These effector T cells then leave the lymph node, enter the blood, and travel to the area of the body where the invaders they can kill are located. When an effector T cell reaches the battle site, it exits the blood, and begins to hack away at infected cells. Most killing by CTLs requires contact between the CTL and its target cell, and CTLs have several weapons they can use during this "hand-to-hand" combat.

One weapon CTLs employ involves the production of a protein called **perforin**. Perforin is a close relative of the C9 complement protein that is part of the membrane attack complex. Like its cousin, perforin can bind to cell membranes and drill holes in them. For this to happen, a killer T cell's TCRs must first identify the target. Then adhesion molecules on the CTL hold the target cell close while the killer cell delivers a mixture of perforin and an enzyme called **granzyme B** onto the surface of the target cell. Perforin damages the cell's outer membrane, and when the cell tries to repair this damage, both granzyme B and perforin are taken into the cell in a vesicle made from the target cell's membrane. Once inside the target cell, the perforin molecules make holes in the entry vesicle, allowing the granzyme B to escape into the cytoplasm of the cell. So **perforin helps a CTL deliver granzyme B into the cytoplasm of its target cell.** There, granzyme B triggers an enzymatic chain reaction which causes the cell to commit suicide by **apoptosis**. This kind of "assisted suicide" usually involves the destruction of the target cell's DNA by the cell's own enzymes. One important feature of this type of killing is that it is "directed": The CTL delivers its lethal cargo right onto the target cell, so that other cells in the area are not damaged during the slaughter.

After a killer T cell has made contact with its target, it only takes about half an hour to kill the cell, and during each attack, the CTL only uses a fraction of its perforin and granzyme B. Consequently, a single killer T cell can execute multiple target cells.

The second way a CTL can kill is by using a protein on its surface called Fas ligand (FasL) which can bind to the Fas protein on the surface of a target cell. When this happens, a suicide program is set in motion within the target cell, and, again, the cell dies by apoptosis. Interestingly, natural killer cells use these same two mechanisms (perforin/granzyme B or FasL) to kill their targets.

It is worth mentioning here that **there actually are two different ways a cell can die: by necrosis or by apoptosis.** Although the end result is the same (a dead cell), the two processes are quite different. Cells usually die by necrosis either as the result of a wound (e.g., a cut or a burn) or when they are killed by an attacking virus or bacterium. **During necrosis, enzymes and chemicals that normally are safely contained within a living cell are released by the dying cell into the surrounding tissues, where they can do real damage.** In contrast, death by apoptosis is much tidier. As a cell dies by apoptosis, its contents are enclosed in little "garbage bags" (vesicles) made from the outer membrane of the dying cell. These vesicles are then eaten and destroyed by nearby macrophages as part of their garbage collecting duty. Consequently, **during apoptosis, the contents of the target cell don't get out into the tissues to cause damage.** So by killing their targets by inducing apoptosis rather than necrosis, CTLs can rid the body of virus-infected cells without causing the collateral tissue damage that would result from necrotic cell death.

There is another reason why triggering cells to die by apoptosis is an especially effective way for killer T cells to destroy virus-infected cells. **When virus-infected cells die by apoptosis, the DNA of unassembled viruses is destroyed along with the target cell's DNA. In addition, DNA or RNA viruses that have reached various stages of assembly within the cell are enclosed in apoptotic vesicles and are disposed of by macrophages. It is this ability to destroy infected cells and the viruses they contain by inducing apoptosis that makes a killer T cell such a potent antiviral weapon.**

REVIEW

In your body, dendritic antigen presenting cells are stationed beneath all surfaces that are exposed to the outside world. By virtue of this geographic location, they can observe an invasion first hand. In fact, the intelligence they acquire at the scene of the battle is complete enough to allow them to formulate a plan of action for the rest of the immune system. This information is gathered in part through the dendritic cell's pattern-recognition receptors, which detect the "signatures" of different types of invaders. Dendritic cells also have receptors which sense the cytokines given off by other immune system cells that are engaged in the battle. In addition, non-immune cells that reside in different areas of the body give off cytokines that imprint the dendritic cell with a regional identity – so it "remembers" where the battle is taking place.

Armed with all this information on the type of invader and the location of the attack, dendritic cells travel to nearby lymph nodes, where they activate T cells. During this process, the game plan is conveyed to helper T cells in the form of co-stimulatory molecules and cytokines expressed by the dendritic cells. This information tells helper T cells which cytokines to make in order to orchestrate the appropriate defense against a particular invader. In a sense, the dendritic cell functions as the coach of the immune system team, while the Th cell performs the duties of quarterback, calling the plays designed by the coach. The dendritic cell is part of the innate immune system. Consequently, the innate system not only determines when the adaptive system should be activated in response to danger, but it also instructs the adaptive system on which weapons to deploy and where to send them.

In response to the instructions delivered by dendritic cells, helper T cells produce combinations of cytokines that mobilize the weapons especially suited to deal with the invader that is attacking at the moment. Although there are many different cytokines a given Th cell can secrete, the best studied combinations are called Th1, Th2, and Th17. Th1 cytokines are especially good at organizing the immune defense against viruses and bacteria which infect human cells. Th2 helper T cells produce a combination of cytokines that is just right for defending against parasites or against bacteria that have breached the intestinal barrier. And Th17 helper T cells secrete cytokines that mobilize the immune system to defend against fungi or extracellular bacteria. Uncommitted Th cells also can be dispatched to the scene of the conflict where, under the influence of battle cytokines, they become committed to secreting a particular cytokine profile. And once a Th cytokine profile has been established, positive and negative feedback tend to lock in this particular profile. Importantly, the cytokines produced by helper T cells have a very short range, so their effects are quite "local." This feature allows the immune system to defend against different types of invaders which attack different parts of the body.

When we are attacked by viruses or bacteria that infect human cells, dendritic cells can activate killer T cells and dispatch them to the area of the body under attack. Killer T cells destroy infected cells by forcing them to commit suicide – a process called apoptosis. When a cell dies by apoptosis, the contents of the cell are enclosed in vesicles which are quickly ingested by nearby macrophages. This garbage disposal system keeps the potentially destructive chemicals and enzymes of the dying cell from getting out into the tissues and doing damage. And it has the great advantage that the pathogens which infected the cell also are packaged up and disposed of.

SUMMARY FIGURE

Here is our final summary figure, showing both the innate and adaptive systems – and the network they form. Can you identify all the players, and do you understand how they interact with each other?

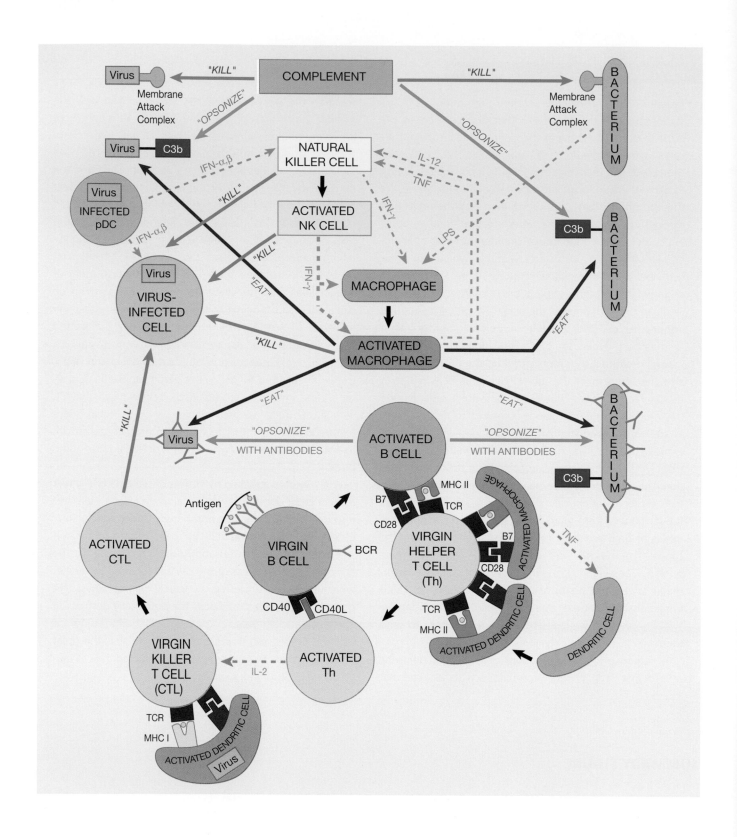

THOUGHT QUESTIONS

1. How does a helper T cell know which cytokine profile to produce?

2. How does a helper T cell "call the plays" for B cells?

3. How does a helper T cell orchestrate the actions of innate system players like macrophages and NK cells?

4. Cytokines have a limited range. Why is this a good thing?

5. What is the difference between death by necrosis and death by apoptosis?

LECTURE 7 | Secondary Lymphoid Organs and Lymphocyte Trafficking

HEADS UP!

The secondary lymphoid organs are strategically placed to intercept invaders which penetrate our barrier defenses. During an infection, rare T cells must find antigen presenting cells that display their cognate antigen, and B cells must encounter helper T cells which can assist them in producing antibodies. The secondary lymphoid organs make it possible for antigen presenting cells, T cells, and B cells to meet under conditions that favor activation. The trafficking of immune system cells throughout our body is controlled by the modulated expression of adhesion molecules on the surface of these cells. Virgin and experienced lymphocytes move in different traffic patterns.

INTRODUCTION

In earlier lectures, we discussed the requirements for B and T cell activation. For example, in order for a helper T cell to assist a B cell in producing antibodies, that Th cells must first be activated by finding an antigen presenting cell which is displaying its cognate antigen. Then the B cell must find that same antigen displayed in a fashion which crosslinks its receptors. And finally, the B cell must find the activated Th cell. When you recognize that the volume of a T or B cell is only about one one-hundred-trillionth of the volume of an average human, the magnitude of this "finding" problem becomes clear. Indeed, it begs the question, "How could a B cell ever be activated?"

The answer is that the movements of the various immune system players are carefully choreographed, not only to make activation efficient, but also to make sure that the appropriate weapons are delivered to the locations within the body where they are needed. Consequently, to really understand how this system works, one must have a clear picture of where in the body all these interactions take place. So it is time now for us to focus on the "geography" of the immune system.

The immune system's defense against an attacker actually has three phases: recognition of danger, production of weapons appropriate for the invader, and transport of these weapons to the site of attack. **The recognition phase of the adaptive immune response takes place in the secondary lymphoid organs. These include the lymph nodes, the spleen, and the mucosal-associated lymphoid tissue (called the MALT for short). You may be wondering: If these are the secondary lymphoid organs, what are the primary ones? The primary lymphoid organs are the bone marrow, where B and T cells are born, and the thymus, where T cells receive their early training.**

LYMPHOID FOLLICLES

All secondary lymphoid organs have one anatomical feature in common: They all contain **lymphoid follicles**. These follicles are critical for the functioning of the adaptive immune system, so we need to spend a little time getting familiar with them. Lymphoid follicles start life as "primary" lymphoid follicles: loose networks of **follicular dendritic cells (FDCs)** embedded in regions of the secondary lymphoid organs that are rich in B cells. So **lymphoid follicles really are islands of follicular dendritic cells within a sea of B cells.**

How the Immune System Works, Fifth Edition. Lauren Sompayrac. © 2016 John Wiley & Sons, Ltd. Published 2016 by John Wiley & Sons, Ltd.

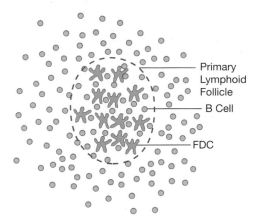

Primary Lymphoid Follicle

B Cell

FDC

Although FDCs do have a starfish-like shape, they are very different from the antigen presenting dendritic cells (DCs) we talked about before. Those dendritic cells are white blood cells that are produced in the bone marrow, and which then migrate to their sentinel positions in the tissues. Follicular dendritic cells are regular old cells (like skin cells or liver cells) that take up their final positions in the secondary lymphoid organs as the embryo develops. In fact, follicular dendritic cells already are in place during the second trimester of gestation. Not only are the origins of follicular dendritic cells and antigen presenting dendritic cells quite different, these two types of starfish-shaped cells have very different functions. Whereas the role of dendritic APCs is to present antigen to T cells via MHC molecules, the function of follicular dendritic cells is to display antigen to B cells. Here's how this works.

Early in an infection, complement proteins bind to invaders, and some of this complement-opsonized antigen will be delivered by the lymph or blood to the secondary lymphoid organs. Follicular dendritic cells that reside in these organs have receptors on their surface which bind complement fragments, and as a result, follicular dendritic cells pick up and retain complement-opsonized antigen. In this way, follicular dendritic cells become "decorated" with antigens that are derived from the battle being waged out in the tissues. Moreover, by capturing large numbers of antigens and by holding them close together, FDCs display antigens in a way that can crosslink B cell receptors. Later during the battle, when antibodies have been produced, invaders opsonized by antibodies also can be retained on the surface of follicular dendritic cells – because FDCs have receptors that can bind to the constant region of antibody molecules.

So follicular dendritic cells capture opsonized antigens and "advertise" these antigens to B cells in a configuration

that can help activate them. Those B cells whose receptors are crosslinked by their cognate antigens hanging from these follicular dendritic "trees" proliferate to build up their numbers. And once this happens, the follicle begins to grow and become a center of B cell development. Such an active lymphoid follicle is called a "secondary lymphoid follicle" or a **germinal center**. The role of complement-opsonized antigen in triggering the development of a germinal center cannot be overemphasized: Lymphoid follicles in humans who have a defective complement system never progress past the primary stage. Thus, we see again that for the adaptive immune system to respond, the innate system must first react to impending danger.

As B cells proliferate in germinal centers, they become very "fragile." Unless they receive the proper "rescue" signals, they will commit suicide (die by apoptosis). Fortunately, helper T cells can rescue these B cells by providing the co-stimulation they need. Indeed, when a B cell whose receptors have been crosslinked by antigen receives this co-stimulatory signal, it is temporarily rescued from apoptotic death, and continues to proliferate.

The rate at which B cells multiply in a germinal center is truly amazing: The number of B cells can double every 6 hours! These proliferating B cells push aside other B cells that have not been activated, and establish a region of the germinal center called the "dark zone" – because it contains so many proliferating B cells that it looks dark under a microscope.

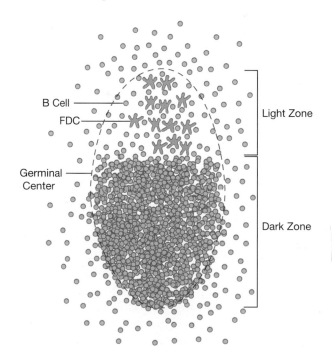

B Cell

FDC

Germinal Center

Light Zone

Dark Zone

After this period of proliferation, some of the B cells "choose" to become plasma B cells and leave the germinal center. Others, during their time of proliferation, undergo somatic hypermutation to fine-tune their receptors. After each round of hypermutation, the affinity of the mutated BCR is tested. Those B cells whose mutated BCRs do not have a high enough affinity for antigen will die by apoptosis, and will be eaten by macrophages in the germinal center. In contrast, B cells are rescued from apoptosis if the affinity of their receptors is great enough to be efficiently crosslinked by their cognate antigen displayed on FDCs – and if they also receive co-stimulation from activated Th cells that are present in the light zone of the germinal center. The current picture is that B cells "cycle" between periods of proliferation and mutation in the dark zone and periods of testing and re-stimulation in the light zone. Sometime during all this action, probably in the dark zone, B cells can switch the class of antibody they produce.

In summary, lymphoid follicles are specialized regions of secondary lymphoid organs in which B cells percolate through a lattice of follicular dendritic cells that have captured opsonized antigen on their surface. B cells that encounter their cognate antigen and receive T cell help are rescued from death. These "saved" B cells proliferate and can undergo somatic hypermutation and class switching. Clearly lymphoid follicles are extremely important for B cell development. That's why all secondary lymphoid organs have them.

HIGH ENDOTHELIAL VENULES

A second anatomical feature common to all secondary lymphoid organs except the spleen is the **high endothelial venule (HEV)**. The reason HEVs are so important is that they are the "doorways" through which B and T cells enter these secondary lymphoid organs from the blood. Most endothelial cells that line the inside of blood vessels resemble overlapping shingles which are tightly "glued" to the cells adjacent to them to prevent the loss of blood cells into the tissues. In contrast, within most secondary lymphoid organs, the small blood vessels that collect blood from the capillary beds (the postcapillary venules) are lined with

special endothelial cells that are shaped more like a column than like a shingle.

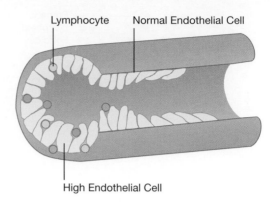

These tall cells are the high endothelial cells. So **a high endothelial venule is a special region in a small blood vessel (venule) where there are high endothelial cells.** Instead of being glued together, high endothelial cells are "spot welded." As a result, there is enough space between the cells of the HEV for lymphocytes to wriggle through. Actually, "wriggle" may not be quite the right term, because lymphocytes exit the blood very efficiently at these high endothelial venules: About 10 000 lymphocytes exit the blood and enter an average lymph node each second by passing between high endothelial cells.

Now that you are familiar with lymphoid follicles and high endothelial venules, we are ready to take a tour of some of the secondary lymphoid organs. On our tour today, we will visit a lymph node, a Peyer's patch (an example of the MALT), and the spleen. As we explore these organs, you will want to pay special attention to the "plumbing." How an organ is connected to the blood and lymphatic systems gives important clues about how it functions.

LYMPH NODES

A lymph node is a plumber's dream. This bean-shaped organ has incoming lymphatics which bring lymph into the node, and outgoing lymphatics through which lymph exits. In addition, there are small arteries (arterioles) that carry the blood that nourishes the cells of the lymph node, and veins through which this blood leaves the node. If you look carefully at this figure, you also can see the high endothelial venules.

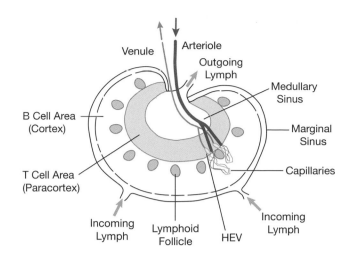

With this diagram in mind, can you see how lymphocytes (B and T cells) enter a lymph node? That's right, they can enter from the blood by pushing their way between the cells of the high endothelial venules. There is also another way lymphocytes can enter the lymph node: with the lymph. After all, lymph nodes are like "dating bars," positioned along the route the lymph takes on its way to be reunited with the blood. And B and T cells actively engage in "bar hopping," being carried from node to node by the lymph. Although lymphocytes have two ways to gain entry to a lymph node, they only exit via the lymph – those high endothelial venules won't let them back into the blood.

Since lymph nodes are places where lymphocytes find their cognate antigen, we also need to discuss how this antigen gets there. When dendritic cells stationed out in the tissues are stimulated by battle signals, they leave the tissues via the lymph, and carry the antigen they have acquired at the battle scene into the secondary lymphoid organs. So this is one way antigen can enter a lymph node: as "cargo" aboard an APC. In addition, antigen which has been opsonized, either by complement or by antibodies, can be carried by the lymph into the node. There the opsonized antigen will be captured by follicular dendritic cells for display to B cells.

When lymph enters a node, it percolates through holes in the marginal sinus (sinus is a fancy word for "cavity"), through the cortex and paracortex, and finally into the medullary sinus – from whence it exits the node via the outgoing lymphatic vessels.

The walls of the marginal sinus are lined with macrophages which capture and devour pathogens as they enter a lymph node. This substantially reduces the number of invaders that the adaptive immune system will

need to deal with. So one of the functions of a lymph node is as a "lymph filter."

The high endothelial venules are located in the paracortex, so B and T cells pass through this region of the node when they arrive from the blood. T cells tend to accumulate in the paracortex, being retained there by adhesion molecules. This accumulation of T cells makes good sense, because dendritic cells also are found in the paracortex – and of course, one object of this game is to get T cells together with these antigen presenting cells. On the other hand, B cells entering a lymph node accumulate in the cortex, the area where lymphoid follicles are located. This localization of B cells works well, because the follicular dendritic cells that display opsonized antigen to B cells are located in this region of the lymph node. So **a lymph node is a highly organized place with specific areas for antigen presenting cells, T lymphocytes, B lymphocytes, and macrophages**.

Lymph node choreography

The fact that different immune system cells tend to hang out in specific places in a lymph node begs the question: How do they know where to go and when to go there? It turns out that the movements of these cells in this secondary lymphoid organ are carefully choreographed by cytokines called **chemokines** (short for chemoattractive cytokines). Here's how this works.

Follicular dendritic cells in a lymph node produce a chemokine called CXCL13. Naive B cells which enter the node express receptors for this chemokine, and are attracted to the area of the node where FDCs are displaying opsonized antigen. If a B cell finds its cognate antigen advertised there, it downregulates expression of the receptors for CXCL13, and upregulates expression of another chemokine receptor, CCR7. This receptor detects a chemokine produced by cells in the region of the lymph node where activated Th cells and B cells meet – the border between the B and T cell areas. Consequently, once a B cell has found its antigen, it is attracted by the "smell" of this chemokine to the correct location to receive help from activated Th cells.

Meanwhile, activated Th cells downregulate expression of the chemokine receptors that have been retaining them in the T cell areas. At the same time, they upregulate expression of CXCR5 chemokine receptors, which cause them to be attracted to the border of the follicle – where antigen-activated B cells are waiting for their help. So **the movement of immune system cells through a lymph node is orchestrated by the up- and downregulation of** chemokine receptors, and the localized production of chemokines that can be detected by these receptors.

Now, of course, human cells don't come equipped with little propellers like some bacteria do, so they can't "swim" in the direction of the source of a chemokine. What human cells do is "crawl." In general terms, the end of the cell that senses the greatest concentration of the chemokine "reaches out" toward the chemokine source, and the other end of the cell is retracted. By repeating this motion, a cell can crawl toward the source of a cytokine.

At this point, you may be asking, "How do activated Th cells know which B cells to help?" It's a good question with an interesting answer. It turns out that when B cells recognize their cognate antigen displayed by follicular dendritic cells, the B cell's receptors bind tightly to this antigen, and the complex of receptor and cognate antigen is taken inside the B cell. So **B cells actually "pluck" antigen from FDC "trees."** Once inside the B cell, the antigen is enzymatically digested, loaded onto class II MHC molecules, and presented on the surface of the B cell for Th cells to see. However, to reach full maturity, B cells that have plucked their antigen need co-stimulation. Activated Th cells can provide this co-stimulation because they express high levels of CD40L proteins that can plug into CD40 proteins on the surface of the B cell. **But Th cells only provide this stimulation to B cells that are presenting the Th cell's cognate antigen.**

Th Cell Helps B Cell

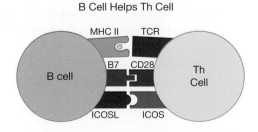

Moreover, Th cells that have been activated by recognizing their cognate antigen also need the assistance of activated B cells in order to mature fully. This assistance involves cell–cell contact during which B7 proteins and proteins called **ICOSL** on the B cell surface bind to CD28 and **ICOS** proteins, respectively, on the Th cell surface.

B Cell Helps Th Cell

What this means is that **at the border of the lymphoid follicle, an activated Th cell and an activated B cell do a "dance" that is critical for their mutual maturation. Th cells provide the CD40L that B cells need. And B cells provide the B7 and ICOSL that helper T cells require for their full maturation. Such fully mature Th cells are called follicular helper T cells (Tfh). These Tfh cells are now "licensed" to rescue fragile, germinal center B cells, and to help these B cells switch classes or undergo somatic hypermutation.**

The initial encounter between Th and B cells generally lasts about 30 minutes, after which some of the B cells proliferate and begin to produce relatively low-affinity IgM antibodies. Although these plasma B cells have not been "upgraded" by class switching or somatic hypermutation, they are important because they provide an immediate antibody response to an invasion. Other B cells and their Tfh partners move together into the germinal center, where class switching and somatic hypermutation can take place. Indeed, **both class switching and somatic hypermutation usually require the interaction between CD40L proteins on Tfh cells and CD40 proteins on the surface of germinal center B cells.**

It is important to note that during this process of bidirectional stimulation, the part of the protein which the B cell recognizes (the B cell epitope) usually is different from the part of the protein that the Th cell recognizes (the T cell epitope). After all, a B cell's receptors bind to the region of a protein which has the right shape to "fit" its receptors. In contrast, a T cell's receptors bind to a fragment of the protein that has the right sequence to fit into the groove of an MHC molecule. Consequently, **although the B cell epitope and the T cell epitope are "linked" – because they come from the same protein – these epitopes usually are different.**

Recirculation through lymph nodes

When a T cell enters a lymph node, it frantically checks several hundred dendritic cells, trying to find one which is presenting its cognate antigen. If a T cell is not successful in this search, it leaves the node and continues to circulate through the lymph and blood. If a helper T cell does encounter a dendritic cell presenting its cognate antigen in the paracortex, the Th cell will be activated and will begin to proliferate. This proliferation phase lasts a few days while the T cell is retained in the lymph node by adhesion molecules. During this time, a T cell can have multiple, sequential encounters with DCs that are presenting its cognate antigen, increasing the T cell's activation level. The expanded population of T cells then leaves the T cell zone. Most newly activated Th cells exit the node via the lymph, recirculate through the blood, and re-enter lymph nodes via high endothelial venules. This process of recirculation is fast – it generally takes about a day – and it is extremely important. Here's why.

There are four major ingredients which must be "mixed" before the adaptive immune system can produce antibodies: APCs to present antigen to Th cells, Th cells with receptors that recognize the presented antigen, opsonized antigen displayed by follicular dendritic cells, and B cells with receptors that recognize the antigen. Early in an infection, there are very few of these ingredients around, and naive B and T cells just circulate through the secondary lymphoid organs at random, checking for a match to their receptors. So the probability is pretty small that the rare Th cell which recognizes a particular antigen will arrive at the very same lymph node that is being visited by the rare B cell with specificity for that same antigen. However, when activated Th cells first proliferate to build up their numbers, and then recirculate to lots of lymph nodes and other secondary lymphoid organs, the Th cells with the right stuff get spread around – so they have a much better chance of encountering those rare B cells which require their help.

B cells also engage in cycles of activation, proliferation, circulation, and re-stimulation. B cells which have encountered their cognate antigen displayed on follicular dendritic cells migrate to the border of the lymphoid follicle where they meet activated T cells that have migrated there from the paracortex. It is during this meeting that B cells first receive the co-stimulation they require for activation. Together, the B and Th cells enter the lymphoid follicles, and the B cells proliferate. Many of the newly made B cells then exit the lymphoid follicle via the lymph. Some become plasma cells that take up residence in the spleen or bone marrow, where they pump out IgM antibodies. Other activated B cells recirculate through the lymph and blood, and re-enter secondary lymphoid organs. As a result, activated B cells are spread around to secondary lymphoid organs where, if they are re-stimulated in lymphoid follicles, they can proliferate more and can undergo somatic hypermutation and class switching.

Killer T cells are activated in the paracortex of the lymph node if they find their cognate antigen presented there by dendritic cells. Once activated, CTLs proliferate and recirculate. Some of these CTLs re-enter secondary lymphoid organs and begin this cycle again, whereas others exit the blood at sites of infection to kill pathogen-infected cells.

As everyone knows, lymph nodes that drain sites of infection tend to swell. For example, if you have a viral infection of your upper respiratory tract (e.g., influenza), the cervical nodes in your neck may become swollen. This swelling is due in part to the proliferation of lymphocytes within the node. In addition, cytokines produced by helper T cells in an active lymph node recruit additional macrophages which tend to plug up the medullary sinuses. As a result, fluid is retained in the node, causing further swelling.

The frenzied activity in germinal centers generally is over in about three weeks. By this time, the invader usually has been repulsed, and a lot of the opsonized antigen has been picked from the follicular dendritic trees by B cells. At this point, most B cells will have left the follicles or will have died there, and the areas that once were germinal centers will look much more like primary lymphoid follicles. And the swelling in your lymph nodes goes away.

When surgeons remove a cancer from some organ in the body, they generally inspect the lymph nodes that drain the lymph from that organ. If they find cancer cells in the draining lymph nodes, it is an indication that the cancer has begun to metastasize via the lymphatic system to other parts of the body – the first stop being a nearby lymph node.

In summary, **lymph nodes act as "lymph filters" which intercept antigen that arrives from infected tissues either alone or as dendritic cell cargo. These nodes provide a concentrated and organized environment of antigen, APCs, T cells, and B cells in which naive B and T cells can be activated, and experienced B and T cells can be re-stimulated. In a lymph node, naive B and T cells can mature into effector cells that produce antibodies (B cells), provide cytokine help (Th cells), and kill infected cells (CTLs). In short, a lymph node can do it all.**

PEYER'S PATCHES

Back in the late seventeenth century, a Swiss anatomist, Johann Peyer, noticed patches of smooth cells embedded in the villi-covered cells that line the small intestine. We now know that these **Peyer's patches** are examples of mucosal-associated lymphoid tissues (MALT) which function as secondary lymphoid organs. Peyer's patches begin to develop before birth, and an adult human has about 200 of them. Here is a diagram that shows the basic features of a Peyer's patch.

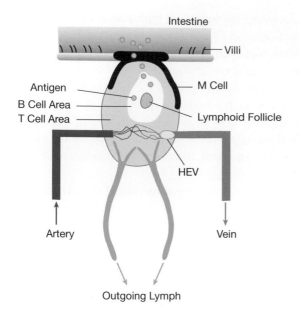

Peyer's patches have high endothelial venules through which lymphocytes can enter from the blood, and, of course, there are outgoing lymphatics that drain lymph away from these tissues. However, unlike lymph nodes, there are no incoming lymphatics that bring lymph into Peyer's patches. So if there are no incoming lymphatics, how does antigen enter this secondary lymphoid organ?

Do you see that smooth cell which crowns the Peyer's patch – the one that doesn't have villi on it? That is called an **M cell**. These remarkable cells are not coated with mucus, so they are, by design, easily accessible to microorganisms that inhabit the intestine. They are "sampling" cells which specialize in transporting antigen from the interior (lumen) of the small intestine into the tissues beneath the M cell. To accomplish this feat, M cells enclose intestinal antigens in vesicles (endosomes). These endosomes are then transported <u>through</u> the M cell, and their contents are spit out into the tissues that surround the small intestine. So, **whereas lymph nodes sample antigens from the lymph, Peyer's patches sample antigens from the intestine – and they do it by transporting these antigens through M cells.**

Antigen that has been collected by M cells can be carried by the lymph to the lymph nodes that drain the Peyer's patches. Also, if the collected antigen is opsonized by complement or antibodies, it can be captured by follicular dendritic cells in the lymphoid follicles that reside beneath the M cells. In fact, except for its unusual method of acquiring antigen, a Peyer's patch is quite similar to a lymph node, with high endothelial venules to admit B and T cells, and special areas where these cells congregate.

Recently it was discovered that M cells are quite selective about the antigens they transport, so M cells don't just take "sips" of whatever is currently in the intestine (how disgusting!). Indeed, these cells only transport antigens that can bind to molecules on the surface of the M cell. This selectivity makes perfect sense. The whole idea of the M cell and the Peyer's patch is to help initiate an immune response to pathogens that invade via the intestinal tract. But for a pathogen to be troublesome, it has to be able to bind to cells that line the intestines and gain entry into the tissues below. So the minimum requirement for a microbe to be dangerous is that it be able to bind to the surface of an intestinal cell. In contrast, most of the stuff we eat will just pass through the small intestine in various stages of digestion without binding to anything. Consequently, by ignoring all the "non-binders," M cells concentrate the efforts of a Peyer's patch on potential pathogens, and help avoid activating the immune system in response to innocuous food antigens.

THE SPLEEN

The final secondary lymphoid organ on our tour is the spleen. This organ is located between an artery and a vein, and it functions as a blood filter. Each time your heart pumps, about 5% of its output goes through your spleen. Consequently, it only takes about half an hour for your spleen to screen all the blood in your body for pathogens.

As with Peyer's patches, there are no lymphatics that bring lymph into the spleen. However, in contrast to lymph nodes and Peyer's patches, where entry of B and T cells from the blood occurs only via high endothelial venules, the spleen is like an "open-house party" in which everything in the blood is invited to enter. Here is a schematic diagram of one of the filter units that make up the spleen.

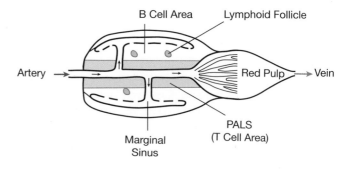

When blood enters from the splenic artery, it is diverted out to the marginal sinuses from which it percolates through the body of the spleen before it is collected into the splenic vein. The marginal sinuses are lined with macrophages that clean up the blood by phagocytosing cell debris and foreign invaders. As they ride along with the blood, naive B cells and T cells are temporarily retained in different areas – T cells in a region called the **periarteriolar lymphocyte sheath (PALS)** that surrounds the central arteriole, and B cells in the region between the PALS and the marginal sinuses.

Of course, since the spleen has no lymphatics to transport dendritic cells from the tissues, you might ask, "Where do the antigen presenting cells in the spleen come from?" The answer is that the marginal sinuses, where the blood first enters the spleen, is home to "resident" dendritic cells. These cells take up antigens from invaders in the blood and use them to prepare a class II MHC display. Resident dendritic cells also can be infected by pathogens in the blood, and can use their class I MHC molecules to display these antigens. Once activated, resident dendritic cells travel to the PALS where T cells have gathered. So although the dendritic cells which present antigens to T cells in the spleen are travelers, their journey is relatively short compared with that of their cousins which travel to lymph nodes from a battle being waged in the tissues.

Helper T cells that have been activated by APCs in the PALS then move into the lymphoid follicles of the spleen to give help to B cells. You know the rest.

THE LOGIC OF SECONDARY LYMPHOID ORGANS

By now, I'm sure you have caught on to what Mother Nature is up to here. **Each secondary lymphoid organ is strategically positioned to intercept invaders that enter the body via different routes.** If the skin is punctured and the tissues become infected, an immune response is generated in the lymph nodes that drain those tissues. If you eat contaminated food, an immune response is initiated in the Peyer's patches that line your small intestine. If you are invaded by blood-borne pathogens, your spleen is there to filter them out and to fire up the immune response. And if an invader enters via your respiratory tract, another set of secondary lymphoid organs that includes your tonsils is there to defend you.

Not only are the secondary lymphoid organs strategically positioned, they also provide a setting that is conducive to the mobilization of weapons that are appropriate to the kinds of invaders they are most likely to encounter. Exactly how this works isn't clear yet. However, it is believed that the different cytokine environments of the various secondary lymphoid organs determine the local character of the immune response. For example, Peyer's patches specialize in turning out Th cells that secrete a Th2 profile of cytokines as well as B cells that secrete IgA antibodies – weapons that are perfect to defend against intestinal invaders. In contrast, if you are invaded by bacteria from a splinter in your toe, the lymph node behind your knee will produce Th1 cells and B cells that secrete IgG antibodies – weapons ideal for defending against those bacteria.

Certainly **the most important function of the secondary lymphoid organs is to bring lymphocytes and antigen presenting cells together in an environment that maximizes the probability that the cells of the adaptive immune system will be activated.** Indeed, the secondary lymphoid organs make it possible for the immune system to react efficiently – even when only one in a million T cells is specific for a given antigen. Earlier, I characterized secondary lymphoid organs as dating bars where T cells, B cells, and APCs mingle in an attempt to find their partners. But in fact, it's even better than that. Secondary lymphoid organs actually function more like "dating services." Here's what I mean.

When men and women use a dating service to find a mate, they begin by filling out a questionnaire that records information on their background and their goals. Then, a computer goes through all these questionnaires and tries to match up men and women who might be compatible. In this way, the odds of a man finding a woman who is "right" for him is greatly increased – because they have been preselected. This type of preselection also takes place in the secondary lymphoid organs.

During our tour, we noted that the secondary lymphoid organs are "segregated," with separate areas for naive T cells and B cells. As the billions of Th cells pass through the T cell areas of the secondary lymphoid organs, only a tiny fraction of these cells will be activated – those whose cognate antigens are displayed by the antigen presenting cells that also populate the T cell areas. The Th cells that do not find their antigens leave the secondary lymphoid organs and continue to circulate. Only those lucky Th cells which are activated in the T cell area will proliferate and then travel to a developing germinal center to provide help to B cells. This makes perfect sense: Allowing useless, non-activated Th cells to enter B cell areas would just clutter things up, and would decrease the chances that

Th and B cells which are "right" for each other might get together.

Likewise, many B cells enter the B cell areas of secondary lymphoid organs, looking for their cognate antigen displayed by follicular dendritic cells. Most just pass on through without finding the antigen their receptors recognize. Those rare B cells which do find their "mates" are retained in the secondary lymphoid organs, and are allowed to interact with activated Th cells. So by "preselecting" lymphocytes in their respective areas of secondary lymphoid organs, Mother Nature insures that when Th cells and B cells eventually do meet, they will have the maximum chance of finding their "mates" – just like a dating service.

LYMPHOCYTE TRAFFICKING

So far, we've talked about the secondary lymphoid organs in which B and T cells meet to do their activation thing, but I haven't said much about how these cells know to go there. Immunologists call this process **lymphocyte trafficking**. In a human, about 500 billion lymphocytes circulate each day through the various secondary lymphoid organs. However, these cells don't just wander around. They follow a well-defined traffic pattern which maximizes their chances of encountering an invader. Importantly, the traffic patterns of virgin and experienced lymphocytes are different. Let's look first at the travels of a virgin T cell.

T cells begin life in the bone marrow and are educated in the thymus (lots more on this subject in Lecture 9). When they emerge from the thymus, virgin T cells express a mixture of cellular adhesion molecules on their surface. These function as "passports" for travel to any of the secondary lymphoid organs. For example, virgin T cells have a molecule called L-selectin on their surface that can bind to its adhesion partner, GlyCAM-1, which is found on the high endothelial venules of lymph nodes. This is their "lymph node passport." Virgin T cells also express an integrin molecule, $\alpha4\beta7$, whose adhesion partner, MadCAM-1, is found on the high endothelial venules of Peyer's patches and the lymph nodes that drain the tissues around the intestines (the mesenteric lymph nodes). So this integrin is their passport to the gut region. Equipped with this array of adhesion molecules, inexperienced T cells circulate through all of the secondary lymphoid organs. This makes sense: The genes for a T cell's receptors are

assembled by randomly selecting gene segments – so there is no telling where in the body a given naive T cell will encounter its cognate antigen.

In the secondary lymphoid organs, virgin T cells pass through fields of antigen presenting cells in the T cell areas. There these T cells check the billboards on several hundred dendritic cells. If they do not see their cognate antigens advertised, they re-enter the blood either via the lymph or directly (in the case of the spleen), and continue to recirculate. Naive T cells make this loop about once a day, spending only about 30 minutes in the blood on each circuit. A naive T cell can continue doing this circulation thing for quite some time, but after about six weeks, if the T cell has not encountered its cognate antigen presented by an MHC molecule, it will die by apoptosis, lonely and unsatisfied. In contrast, those lucky T cells that do find their antigen are activated in the secondary lymphoid organs. These are now "experienced" T cells.

Experienced T cells also carry passports, but they are "restricted passports," because, during activation, expression of certain adhesion molecules on the T cell surface is increased, whereas expression of others is decreased. This modulation of cellular adhesion molecule expression is not random. There's a plan here. In fact, the cellular adhesion molecules that activated T cells express depend on where these T cells were activated. In this way, T cells are imprinted with a memory of where they came from. For example, DCs in Peyer's patches produce retinoic acid which induces T cells activated there to express high levels of $\alpha4\beta7$ (the gut-specific integrin). As a result, T cells activated in Peyer's patches tend to return to Peyer's patches. Likewise, T cells activated in lymph nodes that drain the skin upregulate expression of receptors that encourage them to return to skin-draining lymph nodes. Thus, when activated T cells recirculate, they usually exit the blood and re-enter the same type of secondary lymphoid organ in which they originally encountered antigen. This restricted traffic pattern is quite logical. After all, there is no use having experienced helper T cells recirculate to the lymph node behind your knee if your intestines have been invaded. Certainly not. You want those experienced helper T cells to get right back to the tissues that underlie your intestines to be re-stimulated and to provide help. So by equipping activated T cells with restricted passports, Mother Nature insures that these cells will go back to where they are most likely to re-encounter their cognate antigens – be it in a Peyer's patch, a lymph node, or a tonsil.

Now, of course, you don't want T cells to just go round and round. You also want them to exit the blood at sites of infection. That way CTLs can kill pathogen-infected cells and Th cells can provide cytokines that amplify the immune response and recruit even more warriors from the blood. To make this happen, **experienced T cells also carry "combat passports" (adhesion molecules) which direct them to exit the blood at places where invaders have started an infection.** These T cells employ the same "roll, sniff, stop, exit" technique that neutrophils use to leave the blood and enter inflamed tissues. For example, T cells that gained their experience in the mucosa express an integrin molecule, $\alpha E\beta 7$, which has as its adhesion partner an addressin molecule that is expressed on inflamed mucosal blood vessels. As a result, T cells that have the right "training" to deal with mucosal invaders will seek out mucosal tissues which have been infected. In these tissues, chemokines given off by the soldiers at the front help direct T cells to the battle by binding to the chemokine receptors that appeared on the surface of the T cells during activation. And when T cells recognize their cognate antigen out in the tissues, they receive "stop" signals which tell them to cease migrating and start defending.

In summary, **naive T cells have passports that allow them to visit all the secondary lymphoid organs, but not sites of inflammation. This traffic pattern brings the entire collection of virgin T cells into contact (in the secondary lymphoid organs) with invaders that may have entered the body at any point, and greatly increases the probability that virgin T cells will be activated.** The reason that virgin T cells don't carry passports to battle sites is that they couldn't do anything there anyway – they must be activated first.

In contrast to virgin T cells, **experienced T cells have restricted passports that encourage them to return to the same type of secondary lymphoid organ as the one in which they gained their experience. By recirculating preferentially to these organs, T cells are more likely to be re-stimulated or to find CTLs and B cells that have encountered the same invader and need their help.**

Activated T cells also have passports that allow them to exit the blood at sites of infection, enabling CTLs to kill infected cells and Th cells to provide appropriate cytokines to direct the battle. This marvelous "postal system," made up of cellular adhesion molecules and chemokines, insures delivery of the right weapons to the sites where they are needed.

B cell trafficking is roughly similar to T cell trafficking. **Like virgin T cells, virgin B cells also have passports that admit them to the complete range of secondary lymphoid organs. However, experienced B cells don't tend to be as migratory as experienced T cells. Most just settle down in secondary lymphoid organs or in the bone marrow, produce antibodies, and let these antibodies do the traveling.**

WHY MOTHERS KISS THEIR BABIES

Have you ever wondered why mothers kiss their babies? It's something they all do, you know. Most of the barnyard animals also kiss their babies, although in that case we call it licking. I'm going to tell you why they do it.

The immune system of a newborn human is not very well developed. In fact, production of IgG antibodies doesn't begin until a few months after birth. Fortunately, IgG antibodies from the mother's blood can cross the placenta into the fetus's blood, so a newborn has this "passive immunity" from mother to help tide him over. The newborn can also receive another type of passive immunity: IgA antibodies from mother's milk. During lactation, plasma B cells migrate to a mother's breasts and produce IgA antibodies that are secreted into the milk. This works great, because many of the pathogens a baby encounters enter through his mouth or nose, travel to his intestines, and cause diarrhea. By drinking mother's milk that is rich in IgA antibodies, the baby's digestive tract is coated with antibodies that can intercept these pathogens.

When you think about it, however, a mother has been exposed to many different pathogens during her life, and the antibodies she makes to most of these will not be of any use to the infant. For example, it is likely that the mother has antibodies that recognize the Epstein–Barr virus that causes mononucleosis, but her child probably won't be exposed to this virus until he is a teenager. So wouldn't it be great if a mother could somehow provide antibodies that recognize the particular pathogens that her baby is encountering – and not provide antibodies that the baby has no use for? Well, that's exactly what happens.

When a mother kisses her baby, she "samples" those pathogens that are on the baby's face – the ones the baby is about to ingest. These samples are taken up by the mother's secondary lymphoid organs (e.g., her tonsils), and memory B cells specific for those pathogens are reactivated. These B cells then traffic to the mother's breasts where they produce a ton of antibodies – the very antibodies the baby needs for protection!

In this lecture, we visited three secondary lymphoid organs: a lymph node, a Peyer's patch, and the spleen. Secondary lymphoid organs are strategically situated to intercept invaders that breach the physical barriers and enter the tissues and the blood. Because of their locations, they play critical roles in immunity by creating an environment in which antigen, antigen presenting cells, and lymphocytes can gather to initiate an immune response. To help make this happen, the secondary lymphoid organs are "compartmentalized" with special areas where T cells or B cells are "preselected" before they are allowed to meet.

B and T cells gain access to a lymph node either from the blood (by passing between specialized high endothelial cells) or via the lymph. Antigen can enter a lymph node with lymph drained from the tissues, so this organ functions as a lymph filter that intercepts invaders. In addition, antigen can be carried to a lymph node as cargo aboard an antigen presenting cell. The movement of lymphocytes and dendritic cells within a lymph node is carefully choreographed through the use of cellular adhesion molecules which are up- or downregulated as the cells travel within the node. As a result, helper T cells, which were activated in the T cell areas, move to the boundary of the B cells area to meet with B cells which have recognized their cognate antigen displayed by follicular dendritic cells. There the T and B cells do a "dance" during which the helper T cells become fully "licensed" to help B cells produce antibodies. These licensed Th cells are called follicular helper T cells.

In contrast to a lymph node, antigen is transported into a Peyer's patch through specialized M cells that sample antigen from the intestine. This antigen can interact with B and T cells that have entered the Peyer's patch via high endothelial venules, or it can travel with the lymph to the lymph nodes that drain the Peyer's patch. Thus, a Peyer's patch is a secondary lymphoid organ designed to deal with pathogens which breach the intestinal mucosal barrier.

Finally, we talked about the spleen, a secondary lymphoid organ that is quite different from either a lymph node or a Peyer's patch in that it has no incoming lymphatics and no high endothelial venules. As a result of this "plumbing," antigen and lymphocytes must enter the spleen via the blood. This construction makes the spleen an ideal blood filter that intercepts blood-borne pathogens.

Virgin helper T cells travel though the blood, and enter the secondary lymphoid organs. If a Th cell does not encounter its cognate antigen displayed by an APC in the T cell zone, it exits the organ via the lymph or blood (depending on the organ), and visits other secondary lymphoid organs in search of its cognate antigen. On the other hand, if during its visit to a secondary lymphoid organ, a Th cell does find its cognate antigen displayed by class II MHC molecules on a dendritic cell, it becomes activated and proliferates. Most of the progeny then exit the secondary lymphoid organ and travel again through the lymph and the blood. These "experienced" Th cells have adhesion molecules on their surface that encourage them to re-enter the same type of secondary lymphoid organ in which they were activated (e.g., a Peyer's patch or a peripheral lymph node). This restricted recirculation following initial activation and proliferation spreads activated Th cells around to those secondary lymphoid organs in which B cells or CTLs are likely to be waiting for their help. Recirculating Th cells also can exit the blood vessels that run through sites of inflammation. There Th cells provide cytokines which strengthen the reaction of the innate and adaptive systems to the attack, and which help recruit even more immune system cells from the blood.

Virgin killer T cells also circulate through the blood, lymph, and secondary lymphoid organs. They can be activated if they encounter their cognate antigen displayed by class I MHC molecules on the surfaces of antigen presenting cells in the T cell zones of the secondary lymphoid organs. Like experienced Th cells, experienced CTLs can proliferate and recirculate to secondary lymphoid organs to be re-stimulated, or they can leave the circulation and enter inflamed tissues to kill cells infected with viruses or other parasites (e.g., intracellular bacteria).

Virgin B cells also travel to secondary lymphoid organs, looking for their cognate antigens. If they are unsuccessful, they continue circulating through the blood, lymph, and secondary lymphoid organs until they either find their mates or die of neglect. In the lymphoid follicles of the secondary lymphoid organs, a lucky B cell that finds the antigen to which its receptors can bind will migrate to the border of the lymphoid follicle. There, if it receives the required co-stimulation from an activated helper T cell, the B cell will be activated, and will proliferate to produce many more B cells that can recognize the same antigen. All this activity converts a primary lymphoid follicle, which is just a loose collection of follicular dendritic cells and B cells, into a germinal center in which B cells proliferate and mature. In a germinal center, B cells may class switch to produce IgA, IgG, or IgE antibodies, and they may undergo somatic hypermutation to increase the average affinity of their receptors for antigen. These two "upgrades" usually require the ligation of CD40 on the maturing B cells by CD40L proteins on Tfh cells. Most of these B cells then become plasma cells and travel to the spleen or bone marrow, where they produce antibodies. Others recirculate to secondary lymphoid organs that are similar to the one in which they were activated. There they amplify the response by being re-stimulated to proliferate some more.

THOUGHT QUESTIONS

1. What are the functions of the various secondary lymphoid organs?

2. Make a table for each of the secondary lymphoid organs we discussed (lymph node, Peyer's patch, and spleen) which lists how antigen, B cells, and T cells enter and leave these organs.

3. In the T cell areas of secondary lymphoid organs, activated dendritic cells and Th cells interact. What goes on during this "dance"?

4. At the boundary of the lymphoid follicles of secondary lymphoid organs, B cells and Th cells interact. What goes on during that "dance"?

5. What is the advantage of having virgin T cells circulate through all the secondary lymphoid organs?

6. What is the advantage of having experienced T cells circulate through selected secondary lymphoid organs?

7. Trace the life of a virgin Th cell as it is activated in a lymph node, and eventually makes its way to the tissues of your infected big toe.

Restraining the Immune System

INTRODUCTION

The immune system evolved to provide a rapid and overwhelming response to invading pathogens. After all, most attacks by viruses or bacteria result in acute infections which either are quickly dealt with by the immune system (in a matter of days or weeks) or overwhelm the immune system and kill you. Built into this system are positive feedback loops in which various immune system players work together to get each other fired up. However, once an invasion has been repulsed, these feedback loops must be broken, and the system must be turned off. In addition, there are times when a vigorous response to an invasion simply is not appropriate, and in these situations, the immune system must be restrained in order to prevent irreparable damage to our bodies.

Until recently, immunologists spent most of their effort trying to understand how the immune system gets turned on, and great progress has been made in that area. Now, however, many immunologists have begun to focus on the equally important question of how the system is restrained.

ATTENUATING THE IMMUNE RESPONSE

We generally think of helper T cells as being important in activating the immune system. However, another type of CD4+ T cell has been discovered which actually can dampen the immune response: the inducible regulatory T cell (iTreg). These T cells are termed "inducible" because, just as naive helper T cells can be encouraged to become Th1, Th2, or Th17 cells, naive Th cells activated in an environment that is rich in TGFβ can be "induced" to become iTregs. Inducible regulatory T cells are called "regulatory" because, instead of secreting cytokines such as TNF and IFN-γ, which activate the immune system, iTregs produce cytokines such as IL-10 and TGFβ that help restrain the system.

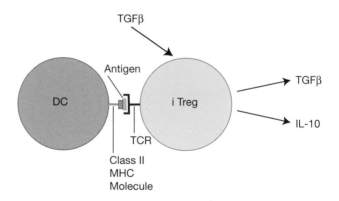

In Lecture 5, we discussed the B7 proteins that are expressed on the surface of antigen presenting cells. These B7 proteins provide co-stimulation to T cells by plugging into receptors called CD28 on a T cell's surface. This interaction sets off a cascade of events within a T cell which reduces the total number of T cell receptors that must be crosslinked in order to activate the T cell – making activation easier. In contrast, the IL-10 secreted by iTreg cells blocks these co-stimulatory signals, and makes it more difficult for APCs to activate naive T cells. In addition, the

TGFβ produced by iTregs reduces the proliferation rate of T cells, and also makes killer T cells less vicious killers. The net result is that iTregs and the cytokines they produce can attenuate the immune response and help keep the system from overreacting.

One area of our body where preventing overexuberance is extremely important is in the tissues that underlie the intestines. Our intestines are home to trillions of harmless bacteria, and inducible regulatory T cells play a major role in keeping the warriors that guard the intestines from overreacting to these bacteria. Intestinal immunity is the subject of Lecture 11.

It also is believed that iTregs are important in protecting us against allergies caused by an overreaction of the immune system to common environmental antigens. In this case, iTregs are thought to act, at least in part, by inhibiting mast cell degranulation – an event which is central to the allergic reaction. We will talk more about allergies in Lecture 13.

DEACTIVATING THE SYSTEM

Even in situations where it is appropriate for the immune system to react strongly against invaders, immune warriors still must be restrained once the battle has been won. During an invasion, as the immune system gains the upper hand and the intruders are destroyed, there will be less and less "invading antigen" present. Consequently, fewer innate system cells will be activated, and fewer dendritic cells will mature and travel with their cargo of battle antigens to secondary lymphoid organs. So **as foreign antigen is eliminated, the level of activation of both the innate and the adaptive system decreases.** This is the first step in turning off the immune system.

Although the removal of foreign antigen is very important, other mechanisms also help decrease the level of activation as the battle winds down. **In addition to engaging stimulatory CD28 molecules on T cells, B7 proteins on APCs also can plug into another receptor on these cells called CTLA-4. In contrast to ligation of CD28, which increases activation, engagement of CTLA-4 represses activation by antagonizing the CD28 signal within the T cell. So ligation of CTLA-4 by B7 proteins acts as a "signal dampener."** Moreover, because B7 binds to CTLA-4 with an affinity thousands of times higher than its affinity for CD28, CTLA-4 also suppresses activation by occupying B7 molecules so they cannot bind to CD28.

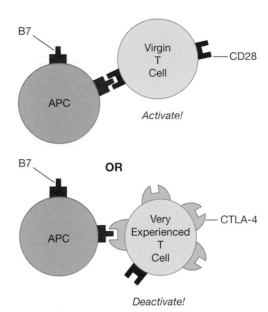

Activate!

OR

Deactivate!

Most human T cells display CD28 on their surface, so it is always available to assist with activation. In contrast, the bulk of a naive T cell's CTLA-4 is stored inside the cell. However, beginning about two days after a virgin T cell is first activated, more and more CTLA-4 is moved from these intracellular reservoirs to the cell surface. There, because of its higher affinity, CTLA-4 eventually out-competes CD28 for B7 binding. As a result, **early in an infection, B7 binds to CD28 and acts as a co-stimulator. Then, after the battle has been raging for a while, B7 binds mainly to CTLA-4. This makes it harder, instead of easier, for these T cells to be reactivated, and helps shut down the adaptive immune response.**

Recently, a molecule with a great name, **programmed death 1 (PD-1)**, has been identified that also helps terminate the immune response. The ligand for PD-1, **PD-1L**, appears on the surface of many different cell types in tissues which are under attack. And like CTLA-4, expression of PD-1 on the T cell surface increases after activation. The result is that the PD-1L protein on inflamed tissues binds to PD-1 on T cells that have been at work for a while, and stops them from proliferating.

In summary, **CTLA-4 functions to make reactivation of T cells less efficient, and PD-1 inhibits the proliferation of previously activated T cells. Together, they function as checkpoint proteins which help "decommission" T cells as the battle winds down.** Unfortunately, ligands for these two molecules also are expressed on cancer cells, and this can limit the ability of T cells to protect against cancer – a subject we will review in more detail in Lecture 15.

LIFE IS SHORT

As a consequence of the removal of foreign antigen and the subsequent cessation of activation, the immune system will stop producing weapons which can defend against a banished invader. Nevertheless, many of the weapons made during the struggle will remain at the battle site, and these stockpiles of obsolete weapons must somehow be eliminated. Fortunately, this problem is partly solved by making many of these weapons short-lived.

During a major invasion, huge numbers of neutrophils are recruited from the blood, but these cells are programmed to die after a few days. Likewise, natural killer cells have a half-life of only about a week. Consequently, once recruitment ceases, the stockpiles of neutrophils and NK cells are quickly depleted. Moreover, because natural killer cells supply IFN-γ to help keep macrophages fired up, when NK cells die off, macrophages tend to go back to a resting state.

Dendritic cells, once they reach a lymph node, only live about a week, and plasma B cells die after about five days of hard labor. Consequently, as the activation of Th and B cells wanes, the number of plasma B cells specific for an invader declines rapidly. In addition, the antibodies which plasma cells produce have short lifetimes, with the longest lived (the IgG class) having a half-life of only about three weeks. As a result, once plasma B cells stop being produced, the number of invader-specific antibodies drops rapidly.

EXHAUSTION

Although many immune system weapons are short-lived, T cells are an important exception to this "rule." In contrast to cells such as neutrophils, which are programmed to self-destruct after a short time on the job, T cells are designed to live a long time. The reason for this is that naive T cells must circulate again and again through the secondary lymphoid organs, looking for their particular antigen on display. Consequently, it would be extremely wasteful if T cells were short-lived. On the other hand, once T cells have been activated, have proliferated in response to an attack, and have defeated the invader, the longevity of T cells could be a major problem. Indeed, at the height of some viral infections, more than 10% of all our T cells recognize that particular virus. If most of these cells were not eliminated, our bodies would soon fill up with obsolete T cells that could only defend us against invaders from the past. Fortunately, Mother Nature recognized this problem and invented **activation-induced cell death (AICD)** – a way of eliminating obsolete T cells after they have been re-stimulated many times in the course of a battle. Here's how this works.

CTLs have proteins called **Fas ligand** that are prominently displayed on their surface, and one way they kill is by plugging this protein into its binding partner, **Fas**, which is present on the surface of target cells. When these proteins connect, the target is triggered to commit suicide by apoptosis. Virgin T cells are "wired" so that they are insensitive to ligation of their own Fas proteins. However, when T cells are activated and then reactivated many times during an attack, their internal wiring changes. During this process, they become increasingly sensitive to ligation of their Fas proteins by their own Fas ligand proteins or by FasL on other T cells. This feature makes these "exhausted" T cells targets for Fas-mediated killing – either by suicide or homicide. By this mechanism, **activation-induced cell death eliminates T cells which have been repeatedly activated, and makes room for new T cells that can protect us from the next microbes which might try to do us in.** In fact, once an invader has been vanquished, more than 90% of the T cells which responded to the attack usually die off.

REVIEW

Inducible regulatory T cells (iTregs) are helper T cells which secrete cytokines designed to keep the immune system "calm" when we are not threatened by dangerous invaders. Also, once a threat has been dealt with, it is important to turn the immune system off, and to dispose of obsolete weapons. The dependence of continued activation on the presence of foreign antigen, and the effect of negative regulators of activation or proliferation such as CTLA-4 and PD-1 help deactivate the system. In addition, the short lifetimes of many immune warriors and the activation-induced death of "fatigued" T cells help reduce the stockpiles of weapons that are no longer needed. These mechanisms combine to "reset" the system after each infection, so that it will be ready to deal with the next attack.

THOUGHT QUESTIONS

1. How do inducible T regulatory cells (iTregs) function to dampen the immune response?

2. Why doesn't the interaction between B7 proteins on APCs and CTLA-4 proteins on naive T cells prevent activation of these T cells?

3. Why do the CTLA-4 and PDL-1 checkpoint proteins work well in combination to help turn off the adaptive immune system late in an infection?

4. Can you imagine why one might want to target CTLA-4 and PDL-1 to help the immune system destroy a cancer?

Self Tolerance and MHC Restriction

HEADS UP!

T cells must be "restricted" to recognize self MHC molecules, so that the attention of these cells will be focused on MHC–peptide complexes, not on unpresented antigen. In addition, T cells and B cells must both be "taught" tolerance, so that they do not attack our own bodies. The safeguards that protect against autoimmunity are multilayered, with each layer designed to catch self-reactive cells that "slip through the cracks" in the layers above. Natural killer cells also are tested to be sure they do not cause autoimmune disease.

INTRODUCTION

The subject of this lecture is one of the most exciting in all of immunology. Part of that excitement arises because, although a huge amount of research has been done on tolerance of self and MHC restriction, there are still many unanswered questions. What really makes this topic so interesting, however, is that it is so important. B cells and T cells must learn not to recognize our own antigens as dangerous. Otherwise we would all die of autoimmune disease.

THE THYMUS

T cells first learn tolerance of self in the thymus, a small organ located just below the neck. This process usually is called **central tolerance induction**. Like the spleen, the thymus has no incoming lymphatics, so cells enter the thymus from the blood. However, in contrast to the spleen, which welcomes anything that is in the blood, entry of cells into the thymus is quite restricted. It is believed that immature T cells from the bone marrow enter the thymus in waves, somewhere in the middle of this organ. However, exactly how this happens is not understood, because the high endothelial cells that allow lymphocytes to exit the blood into secondary lymphoid organs are missing from the thymus.

What is known is that the T cells enter the thymus from the bone marrow "in the nude": They don't express CD4, CD8, or a TCR. After entry, these cells migrate to the outer region of the thymus (the **cortex**) and begin to proliferate.

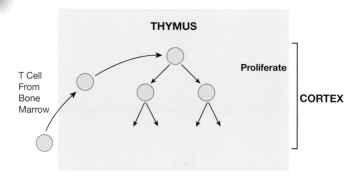

About this time, some of the T cells start to rearrange the gene segments that encode the α and β chains of the TCR. If these rearrangements are successful, a T cell begins to express low levels of the TCR and its associated, accessory proteins (the CD3 protein complex). As a result, the formerly nude T cells soon are "dressed" with CD4, CD8, and TCR molecules on their surface. Because these T cells express both the CD4 and the CD8 co-receptor molecules, they are called **double-positive (DP)** cells.

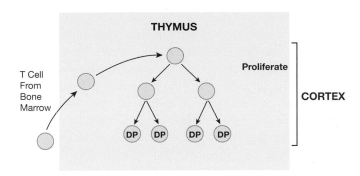

During this "reverse striptease" another important change takes place. When the T cell was naked, it was resistant to death by apoptosis because it expressed little or no Fas antigen (which can trigger cell death when ligated), and because it expressed high levels of Bcl-2 (a cellular protein that protects against apoptosis). In contrast, **a "fully dressed" T cell of the thymic cortex expresses high levels of Fas on its surface and produces very little Bcl-2. Consequently, it is exquisitely sensitive to signals that can trigger death by apoptosis. It is in this highly vulnerable condition that a T cell is tested for MHC restriction and tolerance of self. If it fails either test, it will die a horrible death!**

MHC RESTRICTION

The process of testing T cells for MHC restriction is usually referred to as positive selection. The "examiners" here are epithelial cells in the cortical region of the thymus, and the question a cortical thymic epithelial cell asks of a T cell is: "Do you have receptors that recognize one of the self MHC molecules which I am expressing on my surface?" The correct answer is, "Yes, I do!" for if its TCRs do not recognize any of these self MHC molecules, the T cell dies.

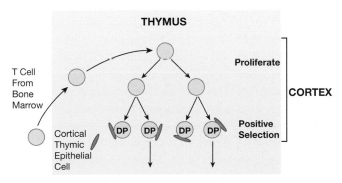

When I say "self" MHC, I simply mean those MHC molecules which are expressed by the person (or mouse)

who "owns" this thymus. Yes, that does seem like a no-brainer – that my T cells would be tested in my thymus on my MHC molecules – but immunologists like to emphasize this point by saying "self MHC."

The MHC molecules on the surface of the cortical thymic epithelial cells actually are loaded with peptides, so **what a TCR really recognizes is the combination of a self MHC molecule and its associated peptide.** The peptides presented by the cortical thymic epithelial cell's class I MHC molecules represent a sampling of the proteins that are being made inside the cell. This is normal class I presentation. Cortical thymic epithelial cells use their class II MHC molecules to present fragments of proteins which they have taken up from the environment within the thymus. This is normal class II MHC presentation. However, immunologists have recently discovered that cortical thymic epithelial cells also employ their class II MHC molecules to present many peptides which don't come from outside these cells. This is what you might called "abnormal" class II MHC presentation. Here's how this works.

Cells have evolved several mechanisms to help them deal with times of famine – situations when the raw materials required for the synthesis of cellular components are limiting. One such survival tool is a process called **autophagy** (literally "self eating"). When cells are starving, they can enclose portions of their cytoplasm in membranes, which then fuse with lysosomes. The cytoplasmic components (e.g., proteins) are then disassembled by lysosomal enzymes so that they can be reused. Remarkably, **cortical thymic epithelial cells also can employ autophagy to capture their own intracellular proteins, digest them into short peptides, and display them on their surface using class II MHC molecules.** By using autophagy to prepare this abnormal display, cortical thymic epithelial cells greatly increase the universe of self peptides they can present to T cells in the thymus. Presumably, this makes it more likely that a T cell will see a combination of a class II MHC molecule and a peptide to which it can bind – and therefore be positively selected for survival.

THE LOGIC OF MHC RESTRICTION

Let's pause for a moment between exams to ask an important question: Why do T cells need to be tested to be sure that they can recognize peptides presented by self MHC molecules? After all, most humans complete their lifetimes without ever seeing "foreign" MHC molecules (e.g., on a transplanted organ), so MHC restriction can't be about discriminating between your MHC molecules and mine. No, MHC restriction has nothing to do with foreign versus self – it's all about focus. As we discussed in Lecture 4, we want the system to be set up so that T cells focus on antigens that are <u>presented</u> by MHC molecules. Like a B cell's receptors, a T cell's receptors are made by mixing and matching gene segments, so they are incredibly diverse. As a result, it is certain that in the collection of TCRs expressed on T cells, there will be many which recognize unpresented antigens, just as a B cell's receptors do. These T cells must be eliminated. Otherwise the wonderful system of antigen presentation by MHC molecules won't work. So the reason positive selection (MHC restriction) is so important is that it sets up a system in which all mature T cells will have TCRs that recognize antigen presented by self MHC molecules.

THYMIC TESTING FOR TOLERANCE OF SELF

During or slightly after positive selection takes place in the cortex of the thymus, T cells stop displaying either one or the other of the co-receptor molecules, CD4 or CD8. As you'd predict, these cells are then called **single positive (SP)** cells. The exact mechanism by which a T cell "chooses" between displaying CD4 or CD8 co-receptors is still being explored. However, the emerging picture is that the choice of co-receptor depends on whether a particular T cell recognizes its cognate antigen displayed by class I or class II MHC molecules on a cortical thymic epithelial cell. For example, if a T cell's receptors recognize an antigen displayed by class I MHC molecules, CD8 co-receptors on the T cell surface will "join the party" and clip onto the MHC molecule. When this happens, the expression of CD4 molecules on that T cell is downregulated. And similarly, a T cell whose receptors recognize a peptide displayed by class II molecules will become a CD4 T cell, and expression of CD8 co-receptors on that cell will be turned off. This strategy works because CD8 co-receptors only bind to class I MHC molecules, and CD4 co-receptors only bind to class II MHC molecules.

Those lucky T cells whose TCRs recognize self MHC plus peptide proceed from the thymic cortex to the central region of the thymus called the **medulla**. It is in the thymic medulla that the second test is administered: the test for tolerance of self. This exam is frequently referred to as **negative selection**.

The exam question asked of T cells during negative selection is: "Do you recognize any of the self peptides displayed by the MHC molecules on my surface?" The correct answer is, "No way!" because T cells with receptors that do recognize the combination of MHC molecules and self peptides are deleted. This second test, which eliminates T cells that could react against our own antigens, is crucial. Indeed, if such self-reactive T cells were not deleted, autoimmune disease could result. For example, Th cells that recognize self antigens could help B cells make antibodies that would tag our own molecules (e.g., the insulin proteins in our blood) for destruction – or CTLs could be produced that would attack our own cells. The latest thinking is that there are two types of cells which pose this second question, and both cell types are different from the cortical thymic epithelial cells that tested T cells for MHC restriction (positive selection).

Medullary thymic epithelial cells

One of the cell types involved in testing T cells for tolerance of self is the **medullary thymic epithelial cell (mTEC)**. These cells are cousins of the cortical thymic epithelial cells that test for MHC restriction, and they have two properties which make them especially suited as "tolerance testers." First, like cortical thymic epithelial cells, mTECs use autophagy to digest their own "innards" and process these proteins for presentation by class II MHC molecules. This rule-breaking presentation, in which proteins made within the cell are displayed by class II MHC molecules, provides a diverse source of self antigens that can be used to eliminate most self-reactive helper T cells during negative selection.

However, there still is a problem. In addition to the "shared" proteins which all cells produce, there are many proteins (estimates suggest several thousand) that are "tissue-specific." These **tissue-specific proteins** are the ones which give each organ or tissue type its identity. For example, there are proteins produced by the cells that make up your heart which are unique to that organ. Also, there are proteins made by kidney cells that are kidney-specific. So for tolerance testing in the thymus to be complete, tissue-specific proteins would need to be included in the "material" on which student T cells are tested. Otherwise, when killer T cells leave the thymus, some of them would surely encounter tissue-specific proteins to which they were not tolerant – and set about destroying your liver, your heart, or your kidneys. Not good.

Recently, it was discovered that medullary thymic epithelial cells produce a transcription factor called **AIRE** that drives expression of many tissue-specific antigens. Consequently, medullary thymic epithelial cells express, in addition to the usual shared proteins, more than a thousand tissue-specific proteins. However, there is still some mystery surrounding the issue of tolerance to tissue-specific antigens. For example, it is not known whether mTECs express all of the tissue-specific proteins found in the body or just most of them.

Thymic dendritic cells

A second cell type has been implicated in testing for tolerance of self antigens in the thymus: the **thymic dendritic cell (TDC)**. Although thymic DCs have the characteristic starfish-like shape, they are different from the dendritic cells we have discussed previously. Some TDCs are "residents" of the thymus which develop there from bone marrow-derived precursors. These dendritic cells are expected to present self antigens which they acquire in the thymus. Other "migratory" TDCs travel to the thymus from various parts of the body where they are thought to capture self antigens for presentation. So far, the relative importance of mTECs and TDCs in tolerance induction is not known. In fact, it isn't even clear whether mTECs actually do the testing, or whether they somehow "hand off" their antigens to TDCs – which then function as the testers. So there is a lot still to be discovered about negative selection in the thymus.

GRADUATION

The final result of all this testing in the thymus is a collection of T cells that have receptors which <u>do</u> recognize self MHC–peptide complexes presented by cortical thymic epithelial cells, but which <u>do not</u> recognize self antigens presented by MHC molecules on thymic dendritic cells or medullary thymic epithelial cells.

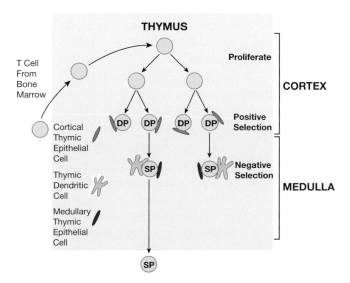

The "thymic graduates" that pass these tests express high levels (i.e., many molecules) of the T cell receptor on their surface, plus either the CD4 or CD8 co-receptor, but not both. Each day in the thymus of a young person, about 60 million double-positive cells are tested, but only about 2 million single-positive cells exit the thymus. The rest die by apoptosis, and are quickly eaten by macrophages in the thymus. Most students are not too thrilled about exams that last more than an hour, so I thought you might like to know that these tests take about two weeks! We're talking major exams here, where the life of each T cell hangs in the balance. Interestingly, immunologists still aren't certain how these graduates leave the thymus, but it is thought that they exit near the corticomedullary junction via the blood.

THE RIDDLE OF MHC RESTRICTION AND TOLERANCE INDUCTION

Now, if you've been paying close attention, you may be wondering how <u>any</u> T cells could possibly pass both exams. After all, to pass the test for MHC restriction, their TCRs must recognize MHC plus self peptide. Yet to pass the tolerance exam, their TCRs must <u>not</u> be able to recognize MHC plus self peptide. Doesn't it seem that the two exams would cancel each other out, allowing no T cells to pass? It certainly does, and this is the essence of the riddle of self tolerance: How can ligation of a T cell receptor possibly result in both positive selection (MHC restriction) and negative selection (tolerance induction)? In fact, it is even more complicated than that, because once a T cell has been educated in the thymus, its TCRs must be able to signal activation when they encounter invader-derived peptides presented by self MHC molecules. So the question that vexes immunologists is: **How does the same TCR, when it engages MHC–peptide complexes, signal three very different outcomes – positive selection, negative selection, or activation?**

Unfortunately, I can't answer this question (otherwise I'd be on my way to Sweden to pick up my Nobel Prize), but I can tell you the current thinking. Immunologists believe that the events leading to MHC restriction and tolerance induction are similar to those involved in the activation of T cells: cell–cell adhesion, TCR clustering, and co-stimulation. It is hypothesized that in the thymus, **positive selection (survival) of T cells results from a relatively weak interaction between TCRs and MHC–self peptide displayed on cortical thymic epithelial cells. Negative selection (death)** is induced by a strong interaction between TCRs and MHC–self peptide expressed on medullary thymic epithelial cells or thymic dendritic cells. And activation of T cells after they leave the thymus results from a strong interaction between TCRs and MHC–peptide displayed by professional antigen presenting cells.

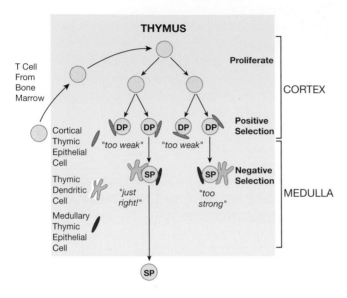

The question, of course, is what makes the effect of these three interactions of MHC–peptide with a T cell receptor so different: life, death, or activation? One key element appears to be the properties of the cell that "sends" the signals. In the case of MHC restriction, this is a cortical thymic epithelial cell. For tolerance induction, the cell is a bone marrow-derived dendritic cell or a medullary thymic epithelial cell. And for activation, the sender is a specialized antigen presenting cell. All these cells are very different, and it is likely that they differ in the cellular adhesion molecules they express and in the number or type of MHC–peptide complexes they display on their surfaces. Such differences in adhesion molecules and MHC–peptide complexes could dramatically influence the strength of the signal that is sent through the T cell receptor. Moreover, the proteasomes of cortical thymic epithelial cells are subtly different from the proteasomes of the cells that are responsible for negative selection. This could affect which self peptides are presented by these examiner cells. In addition, the different types of sender cells are likely to express different mixtures of co-stimulatory molecules – and co-stimulatory signals could change the meaning of the signal that results from TCR–MHC–peptide engagements.

Not only are the cells that send the signals different, the "receiver" (the T cell) also may change between exams. It is known that the number of TCRs on the surface of the T cell increases as the cell is educated, and it is also possible that the "wiring" within the T cell changes as the T cell matures. These differences in TCR density and signal processing could influence the interpretation of signals generated by the three types of sender cells.

Although many of the pieces of the MHC restriction/tolerance induction puzzle have been found, immunologists still have not been able to assemble them into a completely consistent picture. More work is required.

TOLERANCE BY IGNORANCE

Thankfully, most T cells with receptors which could recognize our own proteins are eliminated in the thymus. However, central tolerance induction in the thymus is not foolproof. If it were, every single T cell would have to be tested on every possible self antigen – and that's a lot to ask. The probability is great that T cells with receptors which have a high affinity for those self antigens which are abundant in the thymus will be deleted there. However, T cells whose receptors have a low affinity for self antigens, or which recognize self antigens that are rare in the thymus, are less likely to be negatively selected. They may just "slip through the cracks" of central tolerance induction. Fortunately, the system has been set up to deal with this possibility.

Virgin T cells circulate through the secondary lymphoid organs, but are not allowed out into the tissues. This traffic pattern takes these virgins to the areas of the body where they are most likely to encounter APCs and be activated. However, the travel restriction that keeps virgin T cells out of the tissues also is important in maintaining self tolerance. The reason is that, as a rule, those self antigens which are abundant in the secondary lymphoid organs, where virgin lymphocytes are activated, also are abundant in the thymus, where T cells are tolerized. Therefore, as a result of the traffic pattern followed by virgin T cells, most T cells that could be activated by an abundant self antigen in the secondary lymphoid organs already will have been eliminated by seeing that same, abundant self antigen in the thymus.

Conversely, T cells whose receptors recognize self antigens that are relatively rare in the thymus may escape deletion there. However, these same antigens usually exist at such low concentrations in the secondary lymphoid organs that they do not activate potentially self-reactive T cells. Thus, although rare self antigens are present in the secondary lymphoid organs, and although T cells do have receptors which can recognize them, these T cells usually remain functionally "ignorant" of their presence – because the self antigens are too rare to trigger activation. So lymphocyte traffic patterns play a key role not only in insuring the efficient activation of the adaptive immune system, but also in preserving tolerance of self antigens.

TOLERANCE INDUCTION IN SECONDARY LYMPHOID ORGANS

Although the restricted traffic pattern of naive T cells usually protects them from exposure to self antigens which might activate them, this barrier to activation is not absolute. Occasionally, self antigens that are too rare in the thymus to cause deletion of potentially autoreactive T cells are released into the blood and lymphatic systems (e.g., as the result of an injury which causes tissue damage) in concentrations sufficient to activate previously ignorant T cells. But again, Mother Nature has figured out how to deal with this potential problem.

Until recently, it was thought that the thymus' only role in preventing autoimmunity was the elimination of potentially self-reactive T cells. However, in the last few years, it has become clear that there is an additional thymic function which helps protect us from autoimmune disease – the generation of **natural regulatory T cells (nTregs)**. In the thymus, a subset of CD4+ T cells is selected (by a mechanism that is not well understood) to become natural regulatory T cells. One result of this selection is that these T cells express a gene called **Foxp3**, which is instrumental in conferring upon nTreg cells their regulatory properties. After they are generated in the thymus, natural Tregs receive passports (adhesion molecules) which allow them to enter lymph nodes and other secondary lymphoid organs. Indeed, about 5% of all the CD4+ T cells in circulation are regulatory T cells. If, in a secondary lymphoid organ, a natural Treg encounters its cognate self antigen presented by an antigen presenting cell, it can be activated. Once activated, nTreg cells are able to suppress the activation of potentially self-reactive T cells. Exactly how they accomplish this is still unclear. One likely mechanism is that when a Treg cell recognizes its cognate antigen displayed by an antigen presenting cell, it acts to reduce expression of co-stimulatory molecules on that APC. This makes it more difficult for the APC to activate potentially self-reactive, effector T cells which could recognize that same self antigen.

In the last lecture, you met another type of regulatory T cell: the inducible regulatory T cell. Both inducible and natural regulatory T cells express the Foxp3 protein, but the targets of their suppressive activities appear to be different. Whereas the role of natural regulatory T cells is to provide protection against T cells which have the potential to react against self antigens and cause autoimmunity, the main function of inducible regulatory T cells is to keep the immune system from overreacting to foreign invaders.

Although there is a lot to be discovered about natural Tregs, it is clear that they play an important role in protecting us from autoimmune disease. Indeed, humans who have mutations that compromise the function of the Foxp3 protein suffer from aggressive autoimmune disease and die at an early age.

PERIPHERAL TOLERANCE INDUCTION

Of course, virgin T cells aren't perfect, and some do stray from the prescribed traffic pattern and venture out into the tissues. Indeed, potentially self-reactive T cells are found in the tissues of every normal human. There these "lawbreakers" may encounter self antigens that were too rare in the thymus to trigger deletion, but which are abundant enough in the tissues to activate these T cells. To deal with this situation, there is another level of protection against autoimmunity: **peripheral tolerance induction**.

Because of the two-key requirement for T cell activation, virgin T cells must not only encounter enough presented antigen to cluster their receptors, they must also receive co-stimulatory signals from the cell that is presenting the antigen. That's where activated antigen presenting cells come in. These special cells have lots of MHC molecules on their surface to present antigen, and they also express co-stimulatory molecules such as B7. In contrast, ordinary cells like heart or kidney cells generally don't express high levels of MHC proteins or don't express co-stimulatory molecules, or both. As a result, a virgin T cell with receptors that recognize a kidney antigen could probably go right up to a kidney cell, and not be activated by it. In fact, it's even better than that. When a virgin T cell recognizes its cognate antigen presented on a cell, but does not receive the required co-stimulation, that T cell is "neutered." It looks like a T cell, but it can no longer perform. Immunologists say the cell is **anergized**. In many cases, cells that are anergized eventually die, so peripheral tolerance induction can result in either anergy or death. Consequently, the requirement for the second, co-stimulatory "key" during T cell activation protects us against virgin T cells that venture outside their normal traffic pattern.

TOLERANCE DUE TO ACTIVATION-INDUCED CELL DEATH

Okay, so what if a T cell escapes deletion in the thymus, breaks the traffic laws, and ventures out into the tissues. And suppose that this T cell just happens to find its cognate antigen displayed by MHC molecules at a high enough density to crosslink its receptors on a cell that just happens to be able to provide the co-stimulation required to activate the T cell. What then? Well, all is not lost, because there is yet another "layer" of tolerance induction that can protect us in this unlikely situation.

In the last lecture, we discussed activation-induced cell death (AICD) as one way T cells are eliminated when an invader has been vanquished. This same mechanism also helps protect against virgin T cells that break the traffic rules and are activated by self antigens out in the tissues. T cells in this situation are stimulated over and over by the ever-present self antigens, and when this happens, the self-reactive T cells usually are eliminated by activation-induced cell death. It is as if the immune system senses that this continuous reactivation "ain't natural," and does away with the offending, self-reactive T cells.

So T cell tolerance induction is a multilayered process. Rather than trying to come up with a single mechanism which would test every single T cell for self-reactivity, Mother Nature devised a system with at least five tolerance-inducing mechanisms. This multilayered system insures that, for most humans, autoimmune disease never happens.

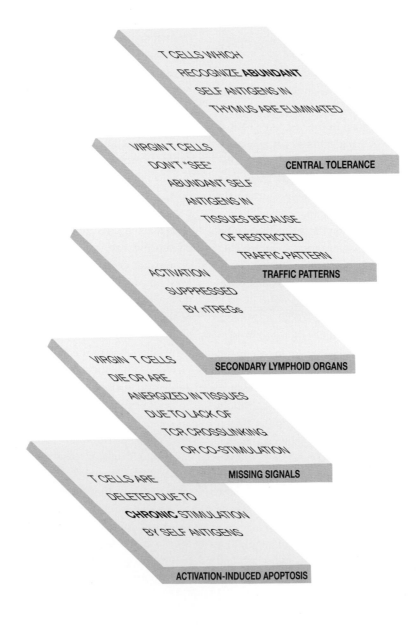

B CELL TOLERANCE

Immunologists once thought that it might not be necessary to delete B cells with receptors that recognize self antigens. The idea was that the T cells needed to help activate potentially self-reactive B cells would already have been killed or anergized. Consequently, B cell tolerance might be "covered" by T cell tolerance. However, it is now clear that mechanisms also exist for tolerizing those B cells which have the potential to be self-reactive.

Most B cells are tolerized where they are born – in the bone marrow. This is the rough equivalent of thymic tolerance induction for T cells. After B cells mix and match gene segments to construct the genes for their receptors, they are "tested" to see if these receptors recognize self antigens that are present in the bone marrow. If a B cell's receptors <u>do</u> recognize a self antigen, it is given another chance to rearrange its light chain genes and come up with new receptors that don't bind to a self antigen. This process is called **receptor editing**, and, in mice, at least 25% of all B cells take advantage of this "second chance." Nevertheless, even when they try again to produce acceptable receptors, only about 10% of all B cells pass the tolerance test. The rest die in the bone marrow.

After testing, B cells with receptors that do not bind to self antigens which are abundant in the bone marrow are released to circulate with the blood and lymph. Of course, induction of B cell tolerance in the bone marrow has the same problems as T cell tolerance induction in the thymus: B cells which have receptors that recognize self antigens that are rare in the marrow can slip through the cracks. Fortunately, bone marrow contains mostly the same abundant self antigens that are found in the secondary lymphoid organs where virgin B cells will be activated. Consequently, **self antigens that are too rare to efficiently delete B cells in the bone marrow usually are too rare to activate these B cells in the secondary lymphoid organs. So the traffic pattern of virgin B cells, which restricts them to circulating through the secondary lymphoid organs, helps protect them from encountering abundant self antigens that are not present in the bone marrow.**

There also are mechanisms which can tolerize B cells that break these traffic laws. For example, **virgin B cells that venture into the tissues can be anergized or deleted if they recognize their cognate antigen but do not receive T cell help.** Thus, B cells are subject to mechanisms which enforce self tolerance out in the tissues that are similar, but not identical, to those which tolerize T cells.

MAINTENANCE OF B CELL TOLERANCE IN GERMINAL CENTERS

In contrast to T cells, which are stuck with the same receptors they express when they are tested in the thymus, B cells have a chance, after they have been activated in the secondary lymphoid organs, to modify their receptors through somatic hypermutation. So you may be wondering whether B cells undergoing somatic hypermutation might end up with receptors that can recognize self antigens. If so, these B cells might produce antibodies that could cause autoimmune disease. Fortunately, it turns out that this usually doesn't happen. Here's why.

If a B cell hypermutates in a germinal center so that its receptors recognize a self antigen, it is very unlikely to find and be stimulated by that self antigen advertised on follicular dendritic cells. After all, FDCs only display antigens that have been opsonized – and self antigens usually aren't opsonized. So the first difficulty that potentially self-reactive B cells face in a germinal center is the lack of opsonized self antigen on follicular dendritic cells. But they have another problem – lack of co-stimulation.

After follicular helper T cells have been activated in the T cell zones of secondary lymphoid organs, they move to the lymphoid follicles to give help to B cells. This help takes place during a dance in which follicular helper T cells (Tfh cells) and B cells stimulate each other. For this co-stimulation to take place, B cells must present the antigen to which their receptors bind to the Tfh cell. Consequently, **for this bidirectional stimulation to work, the Tfh and the B cell must be looking at parts of the same antigen.** If a B cell hypermutates so that its BCRs bind to, internalize, and present a self antigen, that new antigen will not be recognized by the "needy" Tfh cell's receptors. As a result, the B and T cells will not be able to collaborate to keep each other stimulated. They will have lost their "common interest." And because B cells require Tfh cell help to survive in the germinal center, the interdependence of B and Tfh cells keeps B cells "on track" as they undergo somatic hypermutation. So **self tolerance is preserved during B cell hypermutation for two reasons: the lack of opsonized self antigen required for efficient BCR signaling, and the lack of germinal center Tfh cells which can provide help for B cells that recognize self antigen.**

POSITIVE SELECTION OF NATURAL KILLER CELLS

Many viruses try to evade the immune system by down-regulating expression of class I MHC molecules on infected cells. This dirty trick is designed to prevent killer T cells from "looking into" these cells and determining that they are infected. To counter this ploy, natural killer cells survey the cells they come in contact with, and destroy those which do not display class I MHC molecules on their surface – a process called **missing self recognition**. This works because NK cells have "inhibitory receptors" on their surface which recognize class I MHC molecules on healthy cells, and convey a "don't kill" signal. Each NK cell expresses multiple, different inhibitory receptors, and this makes it likely that a given NK cell's inhibitory receptors will recognize at least one of a person's class I MHC molecules. However, inhibitory receptors and class I MHC molecules don't come in "matched pairs." Indeed, a person may have some NK cells whose inhibitory receptors do not recognize any of that person's class I molecules. Such NK cells might conclude that the person's cells were infected – a situation which could be deadly.

To prevent this from happening, NK cells are "examined" to be sure that their inhibitory receptors do recognize at least one of the class I MHC molecules displayed by the cells of the humans they inhabit. NK cells whose inhibitory receptors do not match up with any of a person's class I MHC molecules are rendered non-functional. In this way, NK cells are taught tolerance of self, avoiding NK cell-mediated autoimmunity. The mechanisms involved in this type of "positive selection" are not well understood, but this education is believed to take place in the bone marrow, not in the thymus.

REVIEW

In this lecture, we discussed one of the most important riddles in immunology: How can the same T cell receptor mediate positive selection (MHC restriction), negative selection (tolerance induction), and activation? The current thinking is that in the thymus, positive selection (survival) of T cells whose receptors recognize self MHC results from a relatively weak interaction between TCRs and MHC–self peptides displayed on cortical thymic epithelial cells. This "test" is intended to focus the attention of T cells on antigen presented by MHC molecules, insuring that recognition is restricted to presented antigen, not "native" antigen. Negative selection (death) of cells with TCRs that recognize self antigen in the thymus is induced by a strong interaction between TCRs and MHC–self peptides expressed on medullary thymic epithelial cells or thymic dendritic cells. This "exam" is designed to eliminate T cells which might cause autoimmune disease. Finally, after they leave the thymus, T cells can be activated to defend us against disease through a strong interaction between their TCRs and MHC–peptides displayed by professional antigen presenting cells.

Although thymic (central) tolerance induction is pretty good, it isn't the whole story. One way of dealing with T cells that escape deletion in the thymus is to restrict the trafficking of virgin T cells to blood, lymph, and secondary lymphoid organs. T cells with receptors that recognize antigens which are abundant in the secondary lymphoid organs usually are efficiently deleted in the thymus – where the same antigens also are abundant. Conversely, self antigens that are rare enough in the thymus to allow self-reactive T cells to escape deletion usually are also too rare to activate virgin T cells in the secondary lymphoid organs. Thus, because of their restricted traffic pattern, virgin T cells normally remain functionally ignorant of self antigens that are rare in the thymus.

Natural regulatory T cells in the secondary lymphoid organs also provide protection against autoimmunity, probably by interfering with the activation of potentially self-reactive T cells. And in those cases where virgin T cells do venture outside the blood–lymph–secondary lymphoid organ system, they generally encounter self antigens in a context that leads to anergy or death, not activation. Moreover, those rare T cells that are activated by recognizing self antigens in the tissues usually die from chronic re-stimulation.

Whereas T cells have a separate organ, the thymus, in which central tolerance is induced, B cells with receptors that recognize abundant self antigens are eliminated where they are born – in the bone marrow. During this screening, self-reactive B cells are given a second chance to "edit" their receptors in an attempt to come up with BCRs that do not recognize self antigens.

As with T cells, tolerance induction in B cells is multi-layered. Virgin B cells mainly travel through the blood, lymph, and secondary lymphoid organs. So like T cells, the traffic pattern of naive B cells usually protects them from contact with abundant self antigens on which they were not tested during tolerance induction in the bone marrow. Naive B cells that wander out of the blood/lymph traffic pattern usually don't encounter sufficient self antigen in a form that can crosslink their BCRs. In addition, virgin B cells whose receptors are crosslinked by self antigen in tissues usually don't receive the co-stimulatory signals required for activation – and crosslinking without co-stimulation can anergize or kill B cells.

When B cells mature in germinal centers, they can undergo somatic hypermutation to refine the affinity of their receptors. This process creates the possibility that the mutated BCRs might recognize a self antigen. Fortunately, this usually doesn't happen. In order for B cells to proliferate in germinal centers, their receptors must recognize opsonized antigen displayed by follicular dendritic cells – and self antigens normally are not opsonized. Even more importantly, follicular helper T cells in the germinal center will not recognize the self antigen which the mutated BCRs now recognize and present. And B cells count on help from Tfh cells for survival.

The picture you should have is that none of the mechanisms for tolerizing B and T cells is foolproof – they all are a little "leaky." However, because there are multiple layers of tolerance-inducing mechanisms to catch potentially self-reactive cells, the whole system works very well, and relatively few humans suffer from serious autoimmune disease.

Natural killer cells also are tested to avoid autoreactivity. If an NK cell does not have inhibitory receptors that recognize at least one of a person's class I MHC molecules, that NK cell is rendered non-functional. This process prevents NK cells from attacking healthy cells and causing autoimmunity.

THOUGHT QUESTIONS

1. Why is it important that T cells be tested to be sure they can recognize self MHC molecules? Wouldn't it be a lot simpler just to eliminate this exam?

2. For T cells being educated in the thymus, what is the functional definition of self (i.e., what do these T cells consider to be self peptides)?

3. What is the underlying difficulty in a T cell satisfying both the requirement for MHC restriction (positive selection) and the requirement for tolerance of self (negative selection)?

4. Why are mechanisms needed that can tolerize T cells once they leave the thymus?

5. Explain why the traffic pattern of virgin T cells plays a role in maintaining tolerance of self.

6. Why is it important that B cells also be taught tolerance of self?

7. So far, we have encountered four types of dendritic cells: plasmacytoid dendritic cells, antigen presenting DCs, follicular DCs, and thymic dendritic cells. As a way to review, explain the function of each of these cell types.

LECTURE 10 Immunological Memory

HEADS UP!

The innate immune system has a "hard-wired" memory which allows it to remember encounters with invaders from the ancient past. The adaptive immune system has an "updatable" memory which remembers the specific invaders we have encountered during our lifetime. Memory B and T cells have received "upgrades," and are better able to deal with a second attack than are the B and T cells which responded to the initial invasion.

INTRODUCTION

One of the most important attributes of the immune system is that it remembers past encounters with attackers. These memories help protect against future challenges. Both the innate and the adaptive systems have memories, but what these two systems remember is quite different.

INNATE MEMORY

The innate immune system has a "hard-wired" memory which is extremely important in defending us against everyday invaders. This memory is the result of millions of years of experience, during which the innate system slowly evolved genes for receptors that can detect the signatures of common invaders. These receptors (e.g., Toll-like receptors) usually detect molecular structures which are characteristic of broad classes of microbial pathogens, and which are indispensable for an invader's lifestyle. Moreover, these receptor genes are passed down from generation to generation, and do not change during the lifetime of a human. This ancient memory allows an immediate and robust response to invaders that have been attacking humans for a very long time. Importantly, although the innate immune memory is "tuned" to past invaders, the innate immune system also can protect us against new invaders (for example, viruses that enter the human population from wild animals) if these novel pathogens have structural features in common with ancient invaders.

There is also evidence that some cells of the innate system (e.g., NK cells) can be "trained" by a first exposure to a pathogen to respond more quickly and powerfully to a subsequent invasion by the same type of pathogen. However, this trained memory only seems to work for pathogens that are included in the innate system's "list" of ancient invaders.

ADAPTIVE MEMORY

The innate immune system uses hard-wired receptors to "remember" broad classes of pathogens which also plagued our ancestors (e.g., all those bacteria with LPS as a cell membrane component). In contrast, the adaptive immune system is set up to remember the specific attackers we encounter during our lifetime. Although B and T cells have a diverse collection of receptors that can recognize essentially any invader, there are relatively few naive B or T cells with receptors that can recognize any particular attacker – not enough to mount an immediate defense. So in practical terms, B and T cells really begin life with a blank memory. During an initial attack, pathogen-specific B or T cells proliferate to build up their numbers. Then, when the invader has been subdued, most of these cells die off, but some (typically a few percent) remain as memory B

How the Immune System Works, Fifth Edition. Lauren Sompayrac. © 2016 John Wiley & Sons, Ltd. Published 2016 by John Wiley & Sons, Ltd.

or T cells to defend against a subsequent attack by the same invader.

B cell memory

It is clear that antibodies can confer life-long immunity to infection. For example, in 1781, Swedish traders brought the measles virus to the isolated Faroe Islands. In 1846, when another ship carrying sailors infected with measles visited the islands, most people who were older than 64 years did not contract the disease – because they still had antibodies against the measles virus. Even the longest lived antibodies (the IgG class) have a half-life of less than a month, so antibodies would have to be made continuously over a period of many years to provide this long-lasting protection.

When B cells are activated during the initial response to an invader, three kinds of B cells are generated. First, **short-lived plasma B cells** are produced in the lymphoid follicles of secondary lymphoid organs. These cells travel to the bone marrow or spleen and produce huge quantities of antibodies that are specific for the attacker. Although they only live for a few days, short-lived plasma B cells produce antibodies which are extremely important in protecting us against an enemy that the immune system has never encountered before.

In addition to short-lived plasma B cells, two types of memory B cells are produced in germinal centers during an invasion. Importantly, the generation of both types of memory cells requires T cell help. The first kind of memory B cell is the **long-lived plasma cell**. In contrast to short-lived plasma cells, which are generated rapidly after infection and which die after a few heroic days, long-lived plasma cells take up residence in the bone marrow, and continuously produce more modest amounts of antibodies. It is the long-lived plasma cells which manufacture the antibodies that can provide life-long immunity to subsequent infections. So together, short-lived and long-lived plasma B cells provide both immediate and long-term antibody protection against attacks.

The second type of memory B cell is the **central memory B cell**. These cells reside mainly in the secondary lymphoid organs, and their job is not to produce antibodies. Central memory B cells function as memory "stem cells" which slowly proliferate to maintain a pool of central memory B cells, and to replace long-lived plasma cells which have died of old age. In addition, if another attack occurs, central memory cells can quickly produce more short-lived plasma B cells.

This strategy, which involves three types of B cells, makes good sense. When an invader first attacks, antibodies need to be made quickly to tag invaders for destruction. That's what short-lived plasma B cells do. If, at a later time, the invader attacks again, it is important to already have invader-specific antibodies on hand that can provide an immediate defense. That's the job of long-lived plasma B cells. And between attacks, readiness is maintained by central memory B cells. These cells replenish supplies of long-lived plasma cells and also stand ready to produce a burst of short-lived plasma B cells – cells that can rapidly manufacture large quantities of invader-specific antibodies.

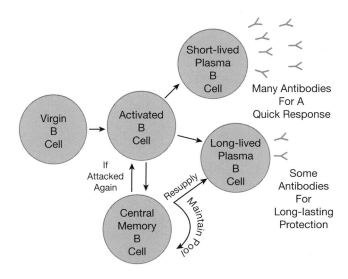

T cell memory

T cells also are able to remember a previous encounter with an invader. Indeed, it has been shown that memory T cells can persist for at least a decade. T cell memory is similar, but not identical, to B cell memory. After naive T cells have been activated in response to an initial attack, and have proliferated to build up their numbers as much as 10 000-fold, many of them are given passports to travel out to the tissues to do battle with the enemy. These are the **effector T cells**. After the attack has been repulsed, about 90% of the effector T cells die by apoptosis, but some of them, the **memory effector T cells**, remain in the tissues near the site of the original encounter with the pathogen. There they wait quietly for a subsequent attack. If that attack comes, they rapidly reactivate, proliferate a bit, and begin to destroy the invaders they remember.

During an attack, some activated T cells do not travel out to the tissues to battle the invaders. They remain in the secondary lymphoid organs. These are the **central memory T cells**. During a subsequent attack, central memory T cells can activate quickly and, after a brief period of proliferation, most mature into effector cells, which join the memory effector T cells at the battle scene. The rest of the central memory T cells remain in the secondary lymphoid organs and wait for another attack by the same invader.

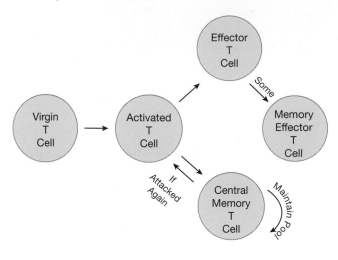

PROPERTIES OF ADAPTIVE MEMORY CELLS

The adaptive immune system remembers specific invaders so well and reacts so powerfully during a subsequent infection that we usually don't even know we have been reinfected. There are a number of reasons why memory cells are better able to deal with a second attack than were the inexperienced B and T cells which responded to the original invasion. First, there are many more of them. Indeed, when we are attacked for the first time, there usually is only about one B or T cell in a million which can recognize that invader. In contrast, by the time the battle is over, the pool of pathogen-specific cells will have expanded so that usually about one in a thousand of all the B or T cells will recognize the attacker. Consequently, the adaptive immune system's response to a subsequent attack is much more robust than the initial response – in part because there are so many more invader-specific cells "on duty."

In addition to being more numerous than their inexperienced predecessors, memory B and T cells are easier to activate. For example, memory T cells can be activated by MHC–peptide concentrations that are as much as 50-fold lower than those required to activate virgin T cells. Also, during the reactivation of memory cells, recognition of

cognate antigen still is required, but at least in some cases, co-stimulation is not essential.

Now why would it be advantageous to have a system in which it is difficult to activate B and T cells the first time, but relatively easy to reactivate them? Clearly, we want activation of virgin cells to be tightly controlled because we only want to engage the adaptive immune system when there is a real threat. Consequently, a fail-safe activation requirement for virgin B and T cells is important. On the other hand, once these cells have been through the stringent two-key selection for primary activation, we want them to respond quickly to a subsequent attack by the same invader – so making it easier for them to be reactivated is a great idea.

There is a third reason why memory B cells are better defenders than are naive B cells: **Memory B cells are "upgraded" versions of the original, virgin B cells.** These upgrades are of two types. First, **during the course of an attack, B cells can switch the class of antibody they make from the "compromise" antibody class, IgM, to one of the other classes (IgG, IgA, or IgE) which specializes in dealing with that particular kind of invader.** This class switch is imprinted on the memory of the B cells that remain after an attack. As a result, memory B cells are able to produce the antibody class which is just right to protect against the invader they remember.

Also, **during an attack, B cells use somatic hypermutation to fine-tune both their receptors and the antibodies they manufacture.** Somatic hypermutation results in upgraded B cell receptors that can detect small amounts of foreign antigen early in an attack. This allows central memory B cells to be activated quickly during a subsequent infection. Somatic hypermutation also results in long-lived plasma cells which make upgraded antibodies that can bind more tightly to the invader.

COMPARING B AND T CELL MEMORIES

B and T cell memories are similar in that both systems center around stem cell-like central memory cells. These central memory cells reside in the secondary lymphoid organs, where they are strategically located to intercept invaders as they enter the body. Memory B and T cells are more potent weapons than are naive cells because a larger fraction of them are specific for the invader they remember, and because they are easier to activate than are virgin B and T cells.

Other aspects of B cell and T cell memory, however, are different. In response to an invasion, B cells can fine-tune their receptors through somatic hypermutation. T cells cannot. Moreover, there is no T cell equivalent of the long-lived plasma B cell. Once we have been exposed to an invader, long-lived plasma B cells continue to produce protective antibodies, frequently for a lifetime. Consequently, the weapons made by B cells (the antibody molecules) continue to be deployed even after an invasion has been repulsed. This works well because antibodies are very specific and rather benign. Only when they tag an invader is the rest of the immune system alerted to take action. So if the invader they recognize doesn't attack again, the antibodies produced by long-lived plasma B cells do nothing and cause no trouble.

In contrast, activated T cells produce cytokines and other chemicals which are non-specific, and which can cause severe damage to normal tissues. Consequently, it would be very dangerous to have T cells remain in action once an invasion has been repulsed. So instead of continuing to function after the enemy has been defeated, as long-lived plasma cells do, effector memory T cells go "dormant." If the attacker does not return, they cause no trouble. On the other hand, if an enemy again enters the tissues where effector memory T cells are "sleeping," these cells quickly reactivate and spring into action.

INNATE VERSUS ADAPTIVE MEMORY

Although both innate and adaptive immune systems remember, it is important to understand how these memories differ. The innate system remembers broad classes of invaders. It does not remember specific invaders. Also, the innate memory is a static memory: It is not updatable – at least not on the time scale of a human lifetime. Although there will be slight genetic differences from human to human, all humans have essentially the same innate memory, which reflects the experience of the human race with common invaders that have been plaguing us for millions of years.

In contrast, the adaptive immune system has an expandable memory that can remember any specific invader to which we have been exposed, be it common or rare. Moreover, the adaptive immune system's memory is personal: Each of us has a different adaptive memory, depending on the particular invaders we have encountered during our lifetime. Not only do we have different "lists" of invaders we have encountered, but even when two people have been attacked by the same microbe, their adaptive memories of that attack will be different – because the receptors on the collection of invader-specific B and T cells will differ from person to person. Indeed, because B and T cell receptors are made by a mix-and-match mechanism, no two humans will have the same adaptive memory.

REVIEW

Both innate and adaptive systems are able to remember past invaders. The innate immune system's memory is hard-wired, and depends on pattern-recognition receptors that have evolved over millions of years to identify common invaders. These receptors recognize signatures which are shared by classes of invaders, and focus on molecular structures that are not easily mutated. In contrast, B and T cells of the adaptive immune system have updatable memories which can remember the individual invaders we have encountered during our lifetimes, both common and rare. Adaptive memory is personal in the sense that every person has a different adaptive memory.

B and T cell memories both require central memory cells which persist in the secondary lymphoid organs following an attack. Central memory T cells react quickly to a second attack by proliferating and maturing into effector T cells, which can travel to the site of the invasion and destroy the enemy. Between attacks, central memory T cells proliferate slowly to maintain a pool of invader-specific T cells.

Central memory B cells also are produced during an attack. If we are invaded again by the same pathogen, central memory B cells quickly activate, proliferate, and most of them mature into plasma B cells – cells which can produce large quantities of pathogen-specific antibodies. Also remaining after a first attack are long-lived plasma B cells which reside in the bone marrow. These cells continuously produce moderate amounts of pathogen-specific antibodies, which give us immediate protection if we are attacked again. This pool of long-lived plasma cells is continually replenished by central memory B cells, which proliferate slowly in the secondary lymphoid organs between invasions.

Memory B and T cells are better able to deal with a second attack because they are much more numerous than before the first invasion, and because they are more easily activated than are virgin B and T cells. Moreover, memory B cells have receptors that have been fine-tuned by somatic hypermutation, and memory B cells usually have class switched to produce the type of antibody molecule which is most appropriate for the invader they remember. As a result of these upgrades, memory B cells are more efficient at dealing with repeat offenders than were their virgin predecessors.

THOUGHT QUESTIONS

1. What are the basic differences between innate system memory and adaptive system memory?

2. What properties of memory B and T cells make them "better, stronger, faster" than the cells which responded to the initial infection?

3. What are the differences between the strategies B and T memory cells use to be sure we are "covered" against a future invasion by the pathogen they remember? Why are these differences important?

4. Why is it that some people appear to have a "good" immune system (i.e., they never get sick), whereas others seem to catch every bug that comes along? Asked another way: Which components of the immune system can differ between individuals?

LECTURE 11

The Intestinal Immune System

HEADS UP!

The intestines are home to trillions of bacteria, some of which "leak" into surrounding tissues. If the intestinal immune system reacts too strongly to these bacteria, intestinal disorders can result. On the other hand, if the immune response is too weak, there is the likelihood of a severe bacterial infection. How does the intestinal immune system know whether to respond gently or forcefully?

INTRODUCTION

One of the most interesting aspects of immunology is that there are still many concepts which are not fully understood – or not understood at all! In this lecture, I want to introduce you to an important area about which there probably are more unknowns than knowns: intestinal immunity. This topic will also give us a chance to review some of the concepts we discussed in earlier lectures.

Most of what is known about the part of the immune system which guards our intestines has been discovered during the last 10 years. Indeed, the gastrointestinal system and its role in human health is currently a hot topic in multiple disciplines. This is because it is now recognized that many diseases such as diabetes, allergies, obesity, some cancers, and inflammatory bowel disease (ulcerative colitis and Crohn's disease) result, at least in part, from an imbalance in the number or type of microbes present in our intestines – or from the immune system's misguided response to these microbes.

The collection of all the microbes (bacteria, viruses, fungi, and parasites) that inhabit our intestines is called the **intestinal microbiota**. By far the most numerous constituents of the intestinal microbiota are the bacteria, and most of the research done to try to understand the interaction between the microbiota and the immune system involves bacteria. Our intestines are home to about 100 trillion bacteria of at least 1000 different types. Most of these are **commensal bacteria** (from the Latin, meaning roughly "to eat at the same table"). Commensals are important for our digestion because they produce enzymes that can break down complex carbohydrates in the food we eat – carbohydrates which cannot be dismantled by the enzymes made by human cells. Some commensal bacteria also produce vitamins that we require for survival. Moreover, because these "friendly" bacteria are so well adapted to live in our intestines, they help protect us from pathogenic bacteria by out-competing the bad guys for available resources and physical niches.

Although commensal bacteria can have a beneficial, symbiotic relationship with their host, they also can be a problem. The single layer of epithelial cells which separates them from the tissues that surround the intestines is so thin, its area so vast, and the bacteria so numerous that, even under normal conditions, some of them will breach this barrier and enter the tissues. In fact, the epithelial "barrier" inhibits, but does not prevent, microbes from entering the tissues that underlie the intestines.

This situation poses a real dilemma. If the intestinal immune system were to react too strongly to commensals, the tissues surrounding your intestines would be in a constant state of inflammation – which would cause diarrhea and all sorts of other problems. On the other hand, if these errant commensal bacteria are not dealt with, they could enter the blood stream and cause a life-threatening, systemic infection. So **the intestinal immune system cannot just ignore commensal bacteria**. Moreover, pathogenic bacteria, which are not so friendly, also can breach the intestinal barrier. In those situations, the immune system must respond appropriately against these dangerous invaders. What this means is that the immune system must somehow decide how to deal gently with intestinal bacteria that are not inherently dangerous, but harshly with those that can do us serious harm. How the immune system tells friend from foe and avoids overreaction is currently the subject of intense investigation.

INTESTINAL ARCHITECTURE

To appreciate what the immune system is up against, we need to have a clear picture of the digestive system and how it works. It is important to note that topologically, our gastrointestinal tract is actually part of the "outside environment." Here is a schematic representation which shows the basic layout.

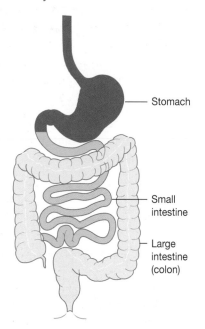

Stomach

Small intestine

Large intestine (colon)

Most of the action, so far as the immune system is concerned, takes place below the stomach in the **small intestine** and the **large intestine (colon)**. The primary function of the small intestine is digestion, and the requirement for absorption of nutrients dictates that the small intestine must have a large area which is separated from the tissues beneath by a single layer of epithelial cells. The small intestine of a human is about 6 meters in length, and its epithelial surface includes millions of finger-like projections called **villi**, which expand the total surface area of the small intestine to nearly 200 square meters.

In contrast, the large intestine is only about 1.5 meters long, has no villi, and plays almost no role in digestion. It has, as its primary function, the reabsorption of water from the intestinal contents. Importantly, the large intestine is home to the vast majority of the commensal bacteria that inhabit the digestive tract.

The **lumen** (i.e., the inside) of both the large and small intestine is bounded by a single layer of epithelial cells. These cells stand shoulder-to-shoulder, are joined together by tight-junction proteins, and are coated with protective **mucus** that is generated by goblet cells in the epithelium. The epithelial cell layer is renewed every three or four days, and it separates the contents of the intestines from the tissues that surround the intestines called the **lamina propria**.

In the small intestine, the mucus is only one layer thick. However, the food and bacteria we ingest move rapidly through the small intestine, so bacteria have to work fast if they are going to get a foothold there. Moreover, the mucus is rich in antibacterial proteins such as lysozyme, which are secreted by cells in the epithelium and which can attack the membranes that surround bacteria. Here is a diagram that shows some of the important features of the small intestine.

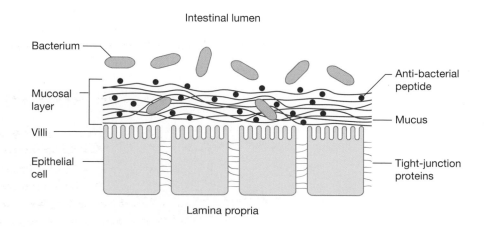

Intestinal lumen

Bacterium

Mucosal layer

Villi

Epithelial cell

Anti-bacterial peptide

Mucus

Tight-junction proteins

Lamina propria

The epithelium of the large intestine is protected by two layers of mucus. The inner layer is firmly attached to the epithelium, and is rather like a pad of steel wool. On top of this dense inner pad is another layer of mucus which, like the single layer in the small intestine, is less dense and more like a slimy net. The layer of mucus closest to the epithelium is relatively bacteria-free, and is rich in antimicrobial peptides (e.g., α-defensins).

The intestinal mucus has several important functions. It acts as a diffusion barrier which denies most of the bacteria in the lumen access to the epithelium. The mucus also concentrates antimicrobial proteins near the epithelial surface – antimicrobials which can destroy bacteria that may try to breach this barrier. These features are important because intestinal infections usually begin when invaders adhere to the epithelial cells that line the intestine. Also, the goblet cells which produce the mucus are hard workers, and the mucus is replaced in a matter of hours. As a consequence, bacteria that are trapped in the mucus are rapidly shown out the "back door" – if you know what I mean.

The mucin proteins that make up the mucus are highly glycosylated. Commensal bacteria feast on these attached carbohydrates, and convert them into short-chain fatty acids such as butyrate and acetate. These molecules easily diffuse through the mucus, and provide an important energy source for the cells of the epithelium.

HOW THE INTESTINAL IMMUNE SYSTEM DEALS WITH INVADERS

Now that we have a clear picture of the intestines, we can discuss how the immune system deals with bacteria which "wander" out of the intestinal lumen into the tissues. One of the defining characteristics of commensal bacteria is that although they may adhere to the epithelium, they do not actively cross this intestinal barrier. Nevertheless, commensals do make their way into the lamina propria as the result of small breaks in the epithelial barrier (no barrier is perfect), and this happens almost continuously. Moreover, after they adhere to the epithelium, some pathogenic bacteria produce virulence factors which allow them to cross the barrier and enter the lamina propria. So the picture you should have is that the intestinal immune system is under constant attack by bacteria and other invaders.

Commensal or pathogenic bacteria which breach the epithelial barrier usually are intercepted by resident macrophages – the most abundant immune system cell in the lamina propria. Invading bacteria also can be transported to nearby mesenteric lymph nodes by the lymphatic vessels that drain the lamina propria. And during an invasion, dendritic cells which reside in the tissues that surround the intestines can travel via the lymphatic route to mesenteric lymph nodes. There they can activate T cells which are specific for the invader, and can encourage these effector cells to travel back to the lamina propria to do battle with the enemy. Indeed, such an inflammatory response is characterized by a dramatic increase in lymphocyte entry into the lamina propria, as well as massive neutrophil recruitment from the blood.

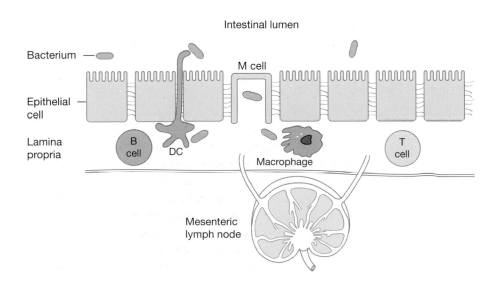

Now if this were all there was to the intestinal immune system, we'd be in big trouble. Commensals are continually breaching the epithelial barrier, so our intestines would be in a state of constant war. Instead of that single splinter in your big toe, this situation would be the rough equivalent of having bacteria-laden splinters piercing the skin all over your body, all the time. It would be awful – and lethal. Clearly, there must be special features of the intestinal immune system which protect us from this sort of overreaction. Let's see what they might be.

Non-inflammatory macrophages

The normal job of macrophages is to cause inflammation. For example, when the tissues beneath the skin are infected with bacteria, macrophages not only phagocytose these invaders, they also secrete cytokines which alert other immune warriors and summon neutrophils from the blood to join in the battle. The result is inflamed tissues at the site of the invasion. In contrast, experiments with mice have shown that special, "non-inflammatory" macrophages patrol the lamina propria. Although these warriors are highly skilled at phagocytosis, they usually do not give off the cytokines which would signal a full-blown attack and cause inflammation. Consequently, **non-inflammatory macrophages can deal gently either with the small number of commensals which continually "leak" from the intestines into the lamina propria, or with a small attack by pathogenic bacteria or viruses.**

IgA antibodies

IgA is the major antibody class produced by B cells in the lamina propria. In fact, **IgA is an antibody designed especially for the protection of mucosal surfaces.** Some of the IgA antibodies produced by lamina propria B cells are transported through the epithelial cells (are "transcytosed") and are released into the lumen of the intestines. **The main task of this "secretory" IgA is exclusion.** Secretory IgA functions by binding to microbes and preventing them from adhering to the epithelial cells that line the intestine. And because the intestinal mucus is renewed frequently, clumps of IgA-bound microbes can be rapidly eliminated with the feces.

Not only can IgA molecules help prevent luminal bacteria from crossing the epithelial barrier, IgA antibodies made by lamina propria B cells also can intercept invaders that have breached the intestinal barrier and have entered the lamina propria. **IgA antibodies in the lamina propria can bind to invaders, transcytose epithelial cells with their cargo, and usher the intruders back out into the intestine for disposal.** Importantly, **secretory IgA does not cause inflam-** mation. This is because the Fc portion of this antibody cannot bind to receptors on immune system cells to trigger an inflammatory response – as, for example, IgG antibodies would do. Consequently, **IgA antibodies can deal gently with intestinal invaders without causing inflammation.**

Although it is not entirely clear how B cells in the lamina propria are influenced to produce IgA antibodies, it is known that retinoic acid given off by intestinal dendritic cells can drive IgA production. Retinoic acid also imprints IgA-secreting plasma B cells with an "intestinal identity," so they home to the tissues that surround the intestines.

In most cases, class switching requires the help of Th cells. This assistance involves the ligation of CD40 on the B cell surface by CD40L on the helper T cell. It appears, however, that B cells of the intestinal immune system also can switch to the production of IgA antibodies without T cell help. It is presumed that other proteins in the intestinal environment can substitute for CD40L, and can ligate the CD40 proteins on intestinal B cells. As I promised, in immunology there is an exception to every rule!

A distributed response

The systemic immune system responds "locally" to, for example, a splinter in your big toe. B and T cells activated in the lymph nodes that drain the toe recirculate through the lymph and blood, and exit the blood stream precisely at the scene of the battle. After all, these weapons are specific for the particular invader that has attacked your big toe today, so it wouldn't be useful to send them to your calf – or even to your little toe. There is nothing going on there. The intestinal immune response is quite different. Although B and T cells might be activated in response to bacteria that entered the lamina propria 1 meter down in your small intestine, those lymphocytes don't return just to that spot. In fact, they are distributed throughout the lamina propria. Why is this, you may ask? Doesn't that seem wasteful?

The answer is that whereas the splinter piercing your toe is a rare event, invasions by the resident bacteria in your intestines are continual. Moreover, although the types of commensals do vary as one goes from the top of the small intestine to the anus, the same commensals are present over long stretches of the intestines. Consequently, **a distributed response, in which B and T cells specific for intestinal invaders are stationed throughout the lamina propria, makes sense.** This distributed response has another important feature. In the big toe example, it takes some time to mobilize the troops that are specific for that invader, and to deliver them to the battleground. In contrast, **the intestinal immune system** is "prepared in advance" to deal with common invaders because lymphocytes and IgA antibodies are already "on site." The result is a lightning fast response that can deal with attackers before they can multiply in the tissues, thereby limiting the amount of inflammation.

A private immune system

Another important feature of the intestinal immune system is that it is "compartmentalized." Under normal conditions, the response to intestinal invaders is separate from the systemic immune system that protects other parts of the body from attack. For example, dendritic cells that are activated in the lamina propria travel to the mesenteric lymph nodes that drain the intestinal tissues – but they do not travel any farther along the chain of lymph nodes. In addition, B and T cells activated in the mesenteric lymph nodes have strict instructions to take up residence in the lamina propria. They do not enter the normal traffic pattern of circulating lymphocytes which would carry them to other parts of the body. In a sense, the intestinal immune system is a "private" immune system. What happens in the intestinal compartment stays in the intestinal compartment.

An anti-inflammatory environment

In contrast to the systemic immune system, where inflammation is the game, the "default option" for the intestinal immune system is anti-inflammatory. Indeed, under normal conditions, the environment surrounding the intestines is heavily biased towards producing a gentle reaction. In Lecture 8, we discussed inducible regulatory T cells – special Th cells whose job is to limit inflammation. It turns out that the lamina propria is home to a large number of these cells. The reason for this is that healthy intestinal epithelial cells produce TGFβ, a cytokine which encourages Th cells that are activated in the intestinal environment to become iTregs. These T cells then give off cytokines such as TGFβ and IL-10, which help "calm down" the mucosal immune system.

In some cases, commensal bacteria contribute directly to help maintain the normally immunosuppressive environment of the lamina propria. For example, as part of their normal metabolism, some commensal bacteria produce butyrate. This short-chain fatty acid influences Th cells in the lamina propria to become regulatory T cells, and butyrate also encourages lamina propria macrophages to deal gently with small bacterial attacks. Likewise, *Bacteroides fragilis*, a commensal bacterium, produces a molecule called polysaccharide A. When Toll-like receptors on helper T cells in the lamina propria detect this polysaccharide, those T cells are instructed to produce IL-10, which dampens inflamation. *Bifidobacterium* is a commensal which is a common constituent of the probiotics many people now take to "promote intestinal health." When the Toll-like receptors of intestinal dendritic cells detect the presence of *Bifidobacterium breve*, those DCs are prompted to produce IL-10 to calm the intestines.

How the intestinal immune system responds to pathogens

Okay, so the intestinal immune system is set up to provide a gentle response to commensal bacteria and to small numbers of pathogens. However, in large numbers, both commensals and pathogenic bacteria can cause damaging infections. So how does the intestinal immune system deal with these dangerous invaders?

In response to serious attacks, Th1 cells can be activated. These helper cells oversee the production of IgG antibodies, and secrete cytokines such as IFN-γ which enhance the killing power of lamina propria macrophages. Also, when helper T cells are activated in an environment that is rich in TGFβ and IL-6, these cells are influenced to become Th17 cells – helper T cells which play an important role in the intestinal immune defense against dangerous attacks.

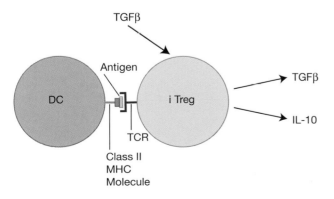

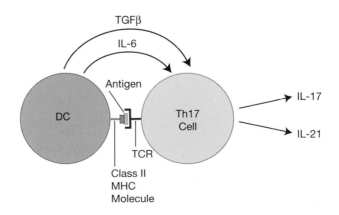

Th17 cells are highly inflammatory. The "signature cytokine" they produce, IL-17, recruits huge numbers of neutrophils from the blood stream – warriors which are just the ticket for dealing with a dangerous bacterial invasion. Cytokines secreted by Th17 cells also function to increase the effectiveness of the intestinal barrier by strengthening the tight junctions between epithelial cells. In addition, these cytokines stimulate mucus production, and act to facilitate the transcytosis of IgA antibodies and their cargo out into the intestinal lumen.

HOW DOES THE INTESTINAL IMMUNE SYSTEM TELL FRIEND FROM FOE?

So the intestinal immune system has the "tools" to deal harshly with dangerous pathogens that invade the digestive tract. But how does the intestinal immune system know to react gently to small doses of commensals or pathogens, and vigorously when there is real danger? For example, TGFβ is a cytokine that drives helper T cells to become iTregs – which are anti-inflammatory. However, TGFβ also is one of the cytokines that causes naive Th cells to become Th17 cells – cells which are skilled at orchestrating an inflammatory response to a bacterial or fungal invasion. So how does the immune system decide whether Th cells should become iTregs and restrain the immune response, or become Th17 cells and "let the dogs out"? The complete answer is unknown. However, as you might predict, **dendritic cells in the lamina propria are thought to play a critical role in maintaining the proper balance between a gentle or an inflammatory response.**

Dendritic cells in the Peyer's patches of the small intestine intercept luminal antigens which have been delivered into the lamina propria by transcytosis through the M cells that crown these patches. In addition, some lamina propria DCs can extend their dendrites between the epithelial cells to make direct contact with antigens in the intestinal lumen. Using these mechanisms, **DCs deliberately and continuously sample what is going on in the intestines, and use this information to decide on an appropriate course of action.**

Dendritic cells are equipped with pattern-recognition receptors that can recognize bacterial "signatures." For example, some of the most pathogenic intestinal bacteria (e.g., *Salmonella*) are equipped with flagella, which help them "swim" through the mucus so they can access the intestinal epithelium. The flagellin protein, from which flagella are constructed, can be detected as a danger signal by TLR5 on the surface of intestinal dendritic cells. And when their Toll-like receptors detect flagellin, DCs begin to produce IL-6, which instructs Th cells to become Th17 cells.

So, if there is no real danger, and things just need to be kept calm, lamina propria DCs don't produce IL-6, and naive Th cells – under the influence of tissue-produced TGFβ – become iTregs. On the other hand, if **there is an invasion of pathogenic bacteria, dendritic cells produce IL-6, which causes helper T cells to commit to becoming Th17 cells.** One important feature of this iTreg to Th17 "switch" is that iTregs are very short lived. Consequently, the switch from suppression to defense can be made quickly.

It is important to note, however, that **commensals and pathogenic bacteria share many of the same molecular features, so in most cases, it is not clear how dendritic cells distinguish between pathogenic and commensal bacteria.** It may be that pathogens and commensals trigger different combinations of pattern-recognition receptors, leading to different outcomes. It also may turn out that the response to pathogens and commensals frequently is the same, and that the decision to respond gently or violently depends on the size of the invasion. In any case, **how the intestinal immune system responds appropriately to intestinal invaders is one of the most important, unsolved mysteries in immunology.** Roughly 1.5 million Americans suffer from Crohn's disease or ulcerative colitis – conditions that are thought to result from an inappropriate inflammatory response to commensal bacteria. So this is an important mystery to solve. Indeed, it is hoped that a better understanding of the intestinal immune system's decision-making process, and how these decisions are implemented, may lead to improved treatments, or even a cure for these diseases.

REVIEW

Trillions of intestinal bacteria are separated from the tissues that surround the intestines by a single layer of epithelial cells covered with mucus. Most of these are commensal bacteria that have evolved a mutually beneficial relationship with their human host. However, there also are pathogenic bacteria which inhabit the intestines, and these can do us serious harm. Both types of bacteria can breach the epithelial barrier, and both must be dealt with by the intestinal immune system.

A variety of immune system defenders, including macrophages, dendritic cells, and lymphocytes, are found beneath the intestinal epithelium in the lamina propria. Under normal conditions, when only small numbers of bacteria leak from the intestines into the lamina propria, these immune warriors operate in an environment which encourages them to deal gently with invaders. Macrophages in the lamina propria normally are non-inflammatory: They are highly phagocytic, but they do not secrete battle cytokines which would "stir up" a full-blown, inflammatory response. B cells in the lamina propria specialize in producing IgA antibodies, which deal passively with invaders by "quietly" transporting them back out into the intestines to be eliminated with the feces. In addition, healthy intestinal epithelial cells produce cytokines which help keep the intestinal immune system relatively calm. These cytokines induce helper T cells to become regulatory T cells, which produce cytokines that have a soothing effect on the immune warriors in the lamina propria.

Dendritic cells in the lamina propria continuously monitor the situation to discover the identity of current invaders. If there is a serious breach of the epithelial barrier, the intestinal immune system can rapidly switch from a gentle response to an aggressive reaction. Alerted dendritic cells can instruct helper T cells to become Th1 or Th17 cells. These helper T cells then orchestrate an inflammatory response in which formerly non-inflammatory macrophages become "angry," and neutrophils are recruited from the blood to engage invaders in hand-to-hand combat.

The weapons of the intestinal immune system are deployed over large areas of the intestines. Because of this distributed response, the intestinal immune system is prepared to deal rapidly with common invaders before they can proliferate to build up their numbers. On the other hand, the intestinal immune system is compartmentalized: Intestinal attacks normally are dealt with locally without spilling over into the rest of the body.

Although some pathogenic bacteria may have unique signatures that alert the intestinal immune system to danger, commensal bacteria and pathogenic bacteria share many of the same molecular features. Consequently, how the intestinal immune system differentiates between friend and foe is one of the important, unsolved mysteries in immunology.

THOUGHT QUESTIONS

1. Discuss several ways in which the intestinal immune system differs from the systemic immune system that protects other areas of the body.

2. What special features of the immune system in the tissues which surround the intestines help avoid an overreaction to commensal bacteria?

3. Why are IgA antibodies called "passive" antibodies?

4. Why are inducible regulatory T cells (iTregs) important, and how do they function?

5. If you were "designing" the intestinal immune system, how would YOU equip it to tell friend from foe? The correct answer to this question might get you a Nobel Prize!

RE 12 | Vaccines

INTRODUCTION

During many "natural" infections, memory B and T cells are generated which can provide protection against a subsequent attack. However, a natural infection can be quite devastating – even lethal. If there was a safe way to trick the immune system into thinking it had been attacked, and to get it to produce memory B and T cells that are appropriate to defend against the anticipated attacker, then a person could be protected against a real infection. That, of course, is what a vaccination does.

A vaccination is the immunological equivalent of the war games our armed forces use to prepare troops for combat. The goal of these "games" is to give soldiers as realistic a simulation of battle conditions as is possible without putting them in great danger. Likewise, a vaccination is intended to prepare the immune system for battle by giving the system as close a look at the real thing as is possible without exposing the vaccine recipient to undue risks. Consequently, the generals who plan war games and the scientists who develop vaccines have a common aim: maximum realism with minimum danger.

Vaccines have been extremely useful in controlling infectious diseases. For example, before a diphtheria vaccine was available, the number of new cases of diphtheria in the United States reached over 350 000 per year. Now, as a result of widespread vaccination against diphtheria, usually fewer than five cases are reported annually.

GENERATING MEMORY HELPER T AND B CELLS

When we are first exposed to an invader, dendritic cells at the battle site ingest the attacker or fragments of the attacker, and travel to nearby lymph nodes. There they use class II MHC molecules to present peptides derived from the invader's proteins. If a helper T cell has receptors which recognize these peptides, it can be triggered to proliferate. Eventually, some of these helper T cells become memory cells which can help protect against a subsequent attack. So for memory helper T cells to be generated, all that is required is for dendritic cells to collect "debris" from the battle scene (e.g., viral coat proteins or part of a bacterial cell membrane) and present peptides derived from this debris to helper T cells.

Likewise, when a B cell's receptors recognize an attacker or a fragment of an attacker which has been transported to the secondary lymphoid organs by the lymph or the blood, that B cell can be activated. After a period of proliferation, if T cell help is available, some of the resulting B cells will become memory cells. So as with helper T cells, even a bit of battle debris is enough to activate a B cell and generate memory B cells. The important point here is that memory B and helper T cells can be produced efficiently even when no immune system cells have been infected by the attacker.

GENERATING MEMORY KILLER T CELLS

Memory killer T cells also can be produced during a microbial attack, but for this to happen, the microbe must infect an antigen presenting cell. For example, if a

How the Immune System Works, Fifth Edition. Lauren Sompayrac. © 2016 John Wiley & Sons, Ltd. Published 2016 by John Wiley & Sons, Ltd.

virus infects a dendritic cell, it will commandeer the cell's biosynthetic machinery, and use it to make viral proteins as part of its reproductive strategy. Some of these proteins will be chopped up into peptides and loaded onto class I MHC molecules. As a result, killer T cells whose receptors recognize the virus' peptides will be activated, and if assistance is available from helper T cells, memory killer T cells will be produced.

So the requirements for generating memory helper T and B cells are different from those for generating memory CTLs. **Memory helper T cells and B cells can be produced even when an invader does not infect an antigen presenting cell. In contrast, for memory killer T cells to be made, the attacker must infect an antigen presenting cell.**

As I mentioned in Lecture 4, under certain experimental conditions, antigen presenting cells can use class I MHC molecules to present antigens taken up from outside the cell. This phenomenon is termed cross-presentation, and it might allow virus-specific CTLs to be generated even when the virus does not infect antigen presenting cells. Currently, the rules that govern cross-presentation are not well understood, and it is not known how important cross-presentation actually is for the normal functioning of the human immune system. Indeed, no antiviral vaccine has been devised that uses cross-presentation to generate protective CTL memory in humans. Of course, it is possible that cross-presentation may eventually be used to produce a vaccine. However, at this time, the rule seems to be that for a vaccine to efficiently generate memory CTLs, antigen presenting cells must be infected. In this lecture, we'll stick to that rule.

STRATEGIES FOR VACCINE DEVELOPMENT

A number of different strategies have been employed to develop the vaccines currently used to protect against microbial infections. In addition, there are innovative, new approaches to vaccine design which are being tested. One important feature of a vaccination is that its efficacy does not depend on the recipient altering his level of hygiene or his lifestyle. Consequently, many believe that a vaccine against HIV-1 may be the best way to stop the spread of AIDS. Because this disease is such an important health issue, as we discuss different types of vaccines, we will ask whether any of them might be suitable to use as a vaccine that would protect against an HIV-1 infection. In the end, I think you will agree that designing a safe and effective AIDS vaccine is a difficult challenge.

A major obstacle to producing an effective AIDS vaccine is that it isn't certain which types of memory cells are needed. The results of trials with vaccines that only produce memory B cells and antibodies suggest that antibodies alone cannot protect against an HIV-1 infection. Indeed, individuals who are infected with HIV-1, but whose immune systems resist the virus for long periods of time, usually have inherited particular class I MHC molecules – suggesting that presentation of antigens to killer T cells is important for resistance. Consequently, most immunologists believe that an effective AIDS vaccine must generate memory killer T cells. Unfortunately, the production of memory CTLs requires that the agent used as a vaccine be capable of infecting antigen presenting cells – and this puts severe restrictions on the types of AIDS vaccines that might be safe to use.

Non-infectious vaccines

Many vaccines are designed not to infect the vaccine recipient. The Salk vaccine for polio is an example of such a "noninfectious" vaccine. To make his vaccine, Dr. Salk treated poliovirus with formaldehyde to "kill" the virus. Formaldehyde acts by gluing proteins together, and the result of this treatment is a virus that looks to the immune system very much like a live poliovirus, but which cannot infect cells because its proteins are non-functional. This treatment is the molecular equivalent of the parking police applying a "boot" to the wheel of a car. The car may look quite normal, but because the wheels can't turn, the vehicle is disabled. The common flu vaccine is a killed virus vaccine, and a similar strategy has been used to make vaccines against disease-causing bacteria. For example, the typhoid vaccine and an effective pertussis (whooping cough) vaccine both are prepared from bacteria that have been grown in the lab and then treated with chemicals such as formaldehyde.

Although the chemicals used to kill these microbes certainly will incapacitate most of them, the procedure is not guaranteed to be 100% effective, and some of them may survive. Now if a vaccine is intended to protect against a virus like influenza, which otherwise will infect a large fraction of the population, the presence of a few live viruses in the vaccine preparation is not a major concern – because without vaccination, many more people would contract the disease. In contrast, if it is intended to protect against a virus such as HIV-1, in which infection is usually preventable (at least for adults in developed countries where blood supplies are carefully screened), a vaccine that has even a small probability of causing the disease could not be used to vaccinate the general public.

Some bacteria produce proteins called toxins that actually cause the symptoms associated with the bacterial infection. In a few cases, these toxins have been used as non-infectious vaccines. To prepare such a vaccine, the toxin is purified and treated with aluminum salts to produce a weakened form of the toxin called a **toxoid**. When injected into a recipient, the toxoid mobilizes B cells that produce antibodies which can bind to and inactivate the harmful toxin during a real attack. Vaccines made from diphtheria or tetanus toxins are examples of this type of non-infectious vaccine.

Non-infectious vaccines also have been prepared by using only certain parts of a pathogen. The idea here is to retain the portions that the immune system needs to see for protection, while discarding the parts that cause unpleasant or dangerous side effects. An "acellular" vaccine for pertussis is made in this way. The original pertussis vaccine was prepared from whole, killed pertussis bacteria, and about half of the infants inoculated with that vaccine had an adverse reaction to it. Fortunately, almost all these side effects were mild when compared with the life-threatening possibility of contracting whooping cough. The acellular vaccine, which has a much lower rate of adverse reactions than the original pertussis vaccine, is made by growing the pertussis bacteria in culture and then purifying several of the bacterial proteins away from the rest of the bacterial components.

Viral proteins produced by genetic engineering also can be used as non-infectious, "subunit" vaccines. The highly effective vaccines against hepatitis B virus and the human papillomavirus are both made in this way. Because only one or a few "synthetic" viral proteins are used to make a subunit vaccine, there is no possibility of infection with the microbe itself (e.g., the hepatitis B virus).

A potential drawback of all non-infectious vaccines is that although they will generate memory helper T cells and B cells (which can make protective antibodies), memory killer T cells will not be made – because antigen presenting cells will not be infected. Of course, many pathogens (e.g., extracellular bacteria) do not infect human cells at all. Consequently, the lack of memory CTLs (which kill infected cells) is not an issue in designing vaccines for these microbes. Also, antibodies produced by memory B cells are sufficient to protect against many pathogens, including some which do infect human cells. For example, poliovirus and hepatitis B virus infect human cells. Nevertheless, the non-infectious Salk poliovirus vaccine and the hepatitis B virus subunit vaccine both work very well – even though neither vaccine generates memory killer T cells. In contrast, killed virus vaccines were unable to protect against either the measles or the mumps virus. So whether memory CTLs are required for protection depends on the particular microbe and its lifestyle.

Attenuated vaccines

Another strategy for producing a vaccine is to use a weakened or "attenuated" form of the microbe. Virologists noticed that when a virus is grown in the laboratory in a cell type which is not its normal host, the virus sometimes accumulates mutations that weaken it. The Sabin polio vaccine, for example, was made by growing poliovirus, which normally reproduces in human nerve cells, in monkey kidney cells. This strategy resulted in polioviruses which were still infectious, but which were so weak they could not cause the disease in healthy individuals. The vaccines for measles, rubella, and mumps, which most children in the United States now receive, are attenuated virus vaccines.

An attenuated vaccine can be tested on animals to get a general idea of whether the attenuation procedure has worked. However, to be sure a crippled microbe can stimulate the production of memory cells, yet not cause disease, it must be tested on humans – usually volunteers who expect to be at risk for contracting the disease. In this regard, it is interesting to note that by the time Dr. Sabin was ready to test his vaccine, most people in the United States had already received the Salk polio vaccine. So at the height of the Cold War, Dr. Sabin took his vaccine to Russia and tested it there. Polio was such a dreaded disease that the Russians were delighted to be "guinea pigs" for Dr. Sabin's made-in-the-USA vaccine.

One important feature of attenuated virus vaccines is that they can produce memory killer T cells. This is because the crippled virus can infect antigen presenting cells and stimulate the production of CTLs before the immune system has had a chance to destroy the weakened invaders. However, because an attenuated vaccine contains a microbe that is infectious, there are safety issues. When a person has recently been vaccinated with an attenuated virus vaccine, he may produce enough virus to infect some of the people with whom he comes in contact. This can be an advantage if those people are healthy, because it spreads the immunity around, producing what immunologists call **herd immunity**. However, a person whose immune system is weakened (e.g., by chemotherapy for cancer) may not be able to subdue the attenuated virus. After all, the attenuated microbe in the vaccine isn't dead. It's just weak. So for those who are immunosuppressed, this type of gratuitous vaccination can have serious consequences.

A second potential safety issue with an attenuated virus vaccine is that before the recipient's immune system subdues the weakened virus, the virus may mutate, and these mutations may restore the strength of the virus. Although this is not a very likely scenario, some healthy people who received the Sabin vaccine have contracted polio because the weakened virus mutated and regained its ability to cause disease.

Carrier vaccines

A relatively new strategy for vaccine preparation uses genetic engineering to introduce a single gene from a pathogenic microbe into a virus that doesn't cause disease. This engineered virus can then be employed as a "Trojan Horse" to carry the gene of the pathogenic microbe into human cells. The idea here is that if the carrier infects the vaccine recipient's antigen presenting cells, these cells will produce the pathogenic microbe's protein as well as the carrier's own proteins. As a result, inoculation with a carrier vaccine should generate memory killer T cells that can protect against a future attack by the real pathogen. Importantly, there is no chance that this vaccine will cause the disease it is designed to protect against – because only one or a few of the pathogen's many genes is "carried" by the vaccine.

It might seem that this approach would be perfect to use to prepare an AIDS vaccine, and vaccines of this type are being tested. Most recently, a vaccine trial in Thailand used a canarypox virus (a cousin of Jenner's cowpox virus) as a Trojan Horse to carry in several genes for HIV-1 proteins. This carrier virus vaccination was then "boosted" by vaccinating the same individuals with a subunit vaccine containing a synthetic version of one of the same HIV-1 proteins produced by the carrier virus. The people receiving these vaccinations, and a roughly equal number of individuals who received a placebo vaccination, were followed for a period of three years to determine how many in each group subsequently became infected with the AIDS virus as a result of risky sexual behavior. Although the authors claimed that the trial "showed a significant, though modest, reduction in the rate of HIV-1 infection," the data is not very convincing. During the study period, 56 people who received the authentic vaccine became infected, whereas 76 members of the group which received the sham vaccine became infected. These are very small numbers on which to

base a meaningful conclusion. Moreover, HIV-specific T cells could only be detected in about 17% of the people who received the vaccine. Finally, when the people who became infected were tested, there was no significant difference in the amount of virus in the blood of members of the two groups. This would suggest that the vaccination had little effect on the ability of infected individuals to resist the viral infection – not what you would expect from an effective vaccine.

VACCINE ADJUVANTS

In order for a vaccine to mimic the invasion of a pathogenic microbe, the immune system must view the vaccine as both foreign and dangerous. This is not a problem for a vaccine which uses a crippled virus – because a crippled virus naturally provides both signals. However, for vaccines composed of only one or a few microbial proteins, providing the requisite danger signal can be a serious problem. Indeed, if a foreign protein is injected into a human, the immune system generally just ignores it because it poses no danger.

Because of this requirement for a danger signal, it is common practice to combine vaccines with an **adjuvant** (derived from a Latin word meaning "help"). In fact, most of the vaccinations you have received probably contained aluminum hydroxide or "alum," which functions, at least in part, by providing that important danger signal. Other, more powerful adjuvants are now being approved for use. For example, the Cervarix vaccine, which can protect against infection by the human papillomavirus, uses MPL, a modified version of the bacterial surface protein LPS, as an adjuvant. In this formulation, viral proteins provide the first signal – specific recognition of something foreign – and MPL alerts the immune system that there is danger associated with these viral proteins. Adding an adjuvant to a vaccine can greatly increase its potency, and can reduce the dose of vaccine which must be administered. Currently, a great deal of research is being carried out to identify powerful adjuvants that are safe for use in humans.

WILL THERE BE AN AIDS VACCINE?

Most immunologists believe that to be effective, an AIDS vaccine must generate memory killer T cells. If true, non-infectious vaccines, which have been used to protect against many other pathogens, will be of little use against HIV-1. In principle, a weakened form of the AIDS virus could be used as a vaccine that would produce memory CTLs. However, because the AIDS virus has an extremely high mutation rate, there is great concern that an attenuated form of HIV-1 might mutate to become lethal again. Consequently, it is very unlikely that a vaccine which uses an attenuated version of the AIDS virus could ever be used to vaccinate the general population. A carrier vaccine could generate memory killer T cells without putting the vaccine recipient at risk for a real AIDS virus infection. So far, however, this strategy has not yielded a vaccine powerful enough to elicit a protective immune response against HIV-1.

Even if a safe vaccine could be devised which would produce HIV-1-specific CTLs, the high mutation rate of the AIDS virus makes it an elusive target. On average, each AIDS virus produced by an infected cell differs from the original infecting virus by at least one mutation. Consequently, the body of someone infected with HIV-1 contains not just "the" AIDS virus, but a huge collection of slightly different HIV-1 strains. As a result, the memory cells produced by a vaccination might protect very well against the particular strain of HIV-1 used to prepare the vaccine, yet be totally useless against other mutant versions of the virus that arise in a real infection. Indeed, the virus' ability to mutate rapidly may prove to be the most difficult problem of all to solve in making an effective AIDS vaccine.

Despite all these difficulties, immunologists are working hard to produce an AIDS vaccine that can be used to protect the public – because such a vaccine is viewed as the current best hope for controlling the spread of the AIDS virus. Recently, antibodies have been discovered in rare AIDS patients which can neutralize many different HIV-1 variants by binding to the virus and preventing it from infecting its target cell. If a vaccine could be made which would elicit these **broadly neutralizing antibodies** in healthy individuals, such a vaccine might be able to protect them from infection – at least by many of the common HIV-1 strains. The plan is to use broadly neutralizing antibodies isolated from patients to identify the site on the virus to which they bind. Then, using this knowledge, it might be possible to devise a synthetic antigen that mimics the structure of this site, and which would elicit broadly neutralizing antibodies in healthy humans. Indeed, this strategy is now being tried with the goal of producing a "universal" vaccine for HIV-1. However, recent experiments with broadly neutralizing antibodies against HIV-1 indicate that these antibodies only arise very late in infection – as the result of many rounds of somatic hypermutation. Whether or not a vaccine can be invented which short-circuits this process and efficiently elicits broadly neutralizing antibodies remains to be seen. Moreover, it may turn out that even broadly neutralizing antibodies are not enough, and that virus-specific CTLs really are required for protection against an HIV-1 infection.

It is important to note that HIV-1 is not the only microbe for which there is no effective vaccine. Roughly two million people die every year from malaria, yet there is no vaccine that has been shown to be generally protective against this disease. Likewise, immunologists have not been able to devise an effective vaccine against tuberculosis, a bacterial infection which kills about three million humans each year. And roughly one third of all the people on earth are infected with herpes simplex virus, yet a herpes vaccine does not exist. Indeed, it is the hope of many that in trying to develop an AIDS vaccine, immunologists will discover new strategies that will make it possible to produce vaccines which will protect against some of the other pathogens for which vaccines currently are not available.

REVIEW

Vaccinations take advantage of the ability of B and T cells to remember invaders we have previously encountered. By introducing the immune system to a "safe" version of a microbe, vaccination prepares these adaptable weapons to respond rapidly and powerfully if a real attack occurs at some future time. The potency of a vaccine can be increased by combining the specific antigen that a B or T cell recognizes together with an adjuvant. The purpose of an adjuvant is to "get the attention of the immune system" by providing a danger signal required for activation.

The production of memory B and helper T cells does not require that an antigen presenting cell be infected.

Consequently, non-infectious vaccines that elicit protective antibodies have been made from dead viruses or even a single viral protein. However, most immunologists believe that to protect against HIV-1 a vaccine will need to elicit memory killer T cells. To do this, a vaccine must be able to infect antigen presenting cells. Attenuated vaccines have been produced using a weakened version of a microbe that can still infect APCs, but cannot cause disease. However, a vaccine intended to protect the general population against HIV-1 must have no possibility of causing AIDS. And because HIV-1 has a very high mutation rate, there are no guarantees that an attenuated AIDS virus will not reactivate. Consequently, an attenuated form of the virus probably cannot be used to protect the public against an HIV-1 infection.

Another approach to making a vaccine that will elicit killer T cell memory is to insert one or more of a microbe's genes into the genome of a benign carrier. Then, when the carrier infects antigen presenting cells, the microbe's proteins will be produced. These proteins can be displayed by class I MHC molecules and can activate CTLs. So far, however, this approach has not produced a generally useful AIDS vaccine.

THOUGHT QUESTIONS

1. Describe the series of events required to produce memory B cells.

2. Describe the series of events required to produce memory CTLs.

3. Compare the advantages and disadvantages of killed virus vaccines and attenuated virus vaccines.

4. What are the major obstacles to producing an AIDS vaccine for the general public?

LECTURE 13

The Immune System Gone Wrong

HEADS UP!

In some situations, the immune system, functioning as intended, can actually make the situation worse. The immune response can be "misguided," mobilizing weapons which are not appropriate to the situation. And in rare instances, the immune system can mistake friend for foe, and attack our own bodies.

INTRODUCTION

Thus far, we have focused on the good that the immune system does in protecting us from infection. Occasionally, however, the immune system "goes wrong" – sometimes with devastating consequences. In this lecture we will examine several situations in which the immune system plays a major role in producing the damaging effects (the pathology) of a disease.

PATHOLOGICAL CONDITIONS CAUSED BY A NORMAL IMMUNE RESPONSE

Tuberculosis is an example of a disease in which the pathology is the unintended consequence of normal immune system function. Tuberculosis is usually contracted by inhaling microdroplets containing the TB bacterium (*Mycobacterium tuberculosis*) that are generated by the cough of an infected individual. When these bacteria are taken into the lungs, they are confronted by macrophages, which are stationed there to intercept invaders that enter via the respiratory tract. A macrophage first engulfs an invader in a phagosome. This

vesicle is then taken inside the macrophage where it fuses with a lysosome that contains powerful chemicals which can destroy most bacteria.

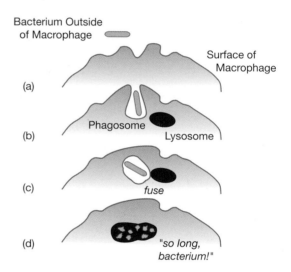

Unfortunately, in the case of the tuberculosis bacterium, the macrophage bites off more than it can chew, because the devious TB bacterium is able to modify the surface of the phagosome so that it does not fuse with the lysosome. Within the phagosome, the bacterium is safe, and it has easy access to all the nutrients it needs to grow and multiply. It is ironic that a TB bacterium happily spends most of its life inside a macrophage – a defender that is supposed to deal harshly with bacterial attackers.

Eventually, many newly minted TB bacteria burst out of the macrophage, killing it. These bacteria then go on to infect other macrophages in the area. As a macrophage dies by necrosis, the contents of its lysosomes are released into the tissues of the lungs. This damages the lungs and initiates an inflammatory reaction which recruits other immune system cells to the battle site, causing even more tissue damage.

The struggle between macrophages and TB bacteria results in the production of battle cytokines that can hyperactivate macrophages in the lungs. Once hyperactivated, the killing power of their weapons increases, so the macrophages can better deal with TB bacteria. However, some of the chemicals given off by hyperactivated macrophages cause additional damage to the tissues of the lungs.

Macrophages and the cells they recruit sometimes win this battle and eliminate the invading bacteria or at least contain them within granulomas. In other cases, it's a fight to a draw, and a state of chronic inflammation results in which the bacteria are kept in check, but macrophages continue to be killed, and the lungs continue to be damaged by the inflammatory reaction. So in a TB infection, the pathology of the disease results from macrophages doing exactly what they are supposed to do – engulf invaders and summon additional immune system cells to help fight the battle.

Sepsis is another disease caused by the immune system trying to do the right thing. Every year, about 250 000 Americans die from sepsis. One important feature of the immune response is that it usually is "local." In fact, our defense system is set up to provide rapid and vigorous responses to numerous small attacks which may come at any point along the boundaries that separate our bodies from the outside world. The aim of this potent local defense is to subdue the enemy quickly before it has a chance to "dig in" and establish its own base of operations. There can be a downside, however, to such a powerful defense: If there is an invasion which is <u>not</u> local, one that affects the whole body, the summation of the potent local immune defenses can actually be life-threatening. Sepsis is a generic term that describes the symptoms which can result from such a systemic infection.

Sepsis usually is caused by bacteria that enter the blood stream when the physical barriers which are our first line of defense are breached. For sepsis to occur in a healthy individual, a large number of bacteria must be introduced into the circulation. This can occur, for example, as a result of bacterial escape from an abscess or other formerly localized infection. In patients with a suppressed immune system (e.g., during chemotherapy for cancer), much smaller quantities of bacteria are required.

Although both Gram-negative and Gram-positive bacteria can cause sepsis, the classic culprits are Gram-negative bacteria like *E. coli* which have lipopolysaccharide (LPS) as a component of their cell membrane. These bacteria also shed this molecule into their surroundings, and LPS is a potent danger signal that can activate macrophages and NK cells. These two cells then cooperate in a positive feedback loop that increases their activation states. Normally, this positive feedback loop amplifies the immune response so that the innate system can respond quickly and strongly to a localized infection. However, in a "full-body" infection in which bacteria carried by the blood enter tissues everywhere, this amplified response can get out of hand. TNF secreted by activated macrophages can cause blood vessels to become "leaky," so that fluid escapes from the vessels into the surrounding tissues. In extreme cases, the decrease in blood volume due to system-wide leakage can cause a drop in blood pressure that results in shock (septic shock) and heart failure. So sepsis and septic shock can result when positive feedback loops, which normally allow the innate immune system to react strongly and quickly, cause an over-reaction to a system-wide infection.

DISEASES CAUSED BY DEFECTS IN IMMUNE REGULATION

Roughly a quarter of the U.S. population suffers from **allergies** to common environmental antigens (**allergens**) that either are inhaled or ingested. Hay fever and asthma are the two most common allergic diseases of the respiratory tract. Hay fever is caused by proteins that are derived from mold spores or plant pollens. These allergens are present in the outside air, usually at certain times of the year. In contrast, the allergens that cause asthma are mostly found indoors. Dust mites, cockroaches, rodents, and household pets are major sources of these allergy-causing proteins. In addition to allergies caused by allergens in the air we breathe, the food we eat also can cause allergies.

The immune systems of non-allergic people respond weakly to these allergens, and produce mainly antibodies of the IgG class. In striking contrast, allergic individuals (called **atopic individuals**) produce large quantities of IgE antibodies. Indeed, the concentration of IgE antibodies in the blood of those with allergies can be 1000- to 10 000-fold higher than that in the blood of non-atopic people! It is the overproduction of IgE antibodies in response to otherwise innocuous environmental antigens that causes allergies.

In Lecture 3, we discussed the interaction of IgE antibodies with white blood cells called **mast cells**. Because mast cell degranulation is a central event in many allergic reactions, let's take a moment to review this concept. When atopic individuals first are exposed to an allergen (e.g., pollen) they produce large amounts of IgE antibodies which recognize that allergen. Mast cells have receptors on their surface that can bind to the Fc region of IgE antibodies. Consequently, after the initial exposure, mast cells will have large numbers of these allergen-specific IgE molecules attached to their surface. Allergens are small proteins with a repeating structure to which many IgE antibodies can bind close together. So on a second or subsequent exposure, an allergen can crosslink the IgE molecules that are bound to the mast cell surface, dragging the mast cell's Fc receptors together. This clustering of Fc receptors tells mast cells to **degranulate**: to release their granules, which normally are stored safely inside the mast cells, into the tissues in which they reside. Mast cell granules contain histamine and other powerful chemicals and enzymes that can cause the symptoms with which atopic individuals are intimately familiar.

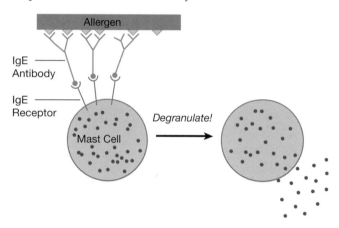

Interestingly, although IgE antibodies have a half-life of only about two days in the blood, once they are attached to mast cells, they have a half-life of weeks to months. This means that mast cells can stay "armed" and ready to degranulate for an extended period after exposure to an allergen.

Allergic reactions generally have two phases: immediate and delayed. The immediate reaction to an allergen is the work of mast cells, which are stationed out in the tissues, and **basophils**, another granule-containing white blood cell, which can be recruited from the blood by signals given off by mast cells responding to an allergen. Like mast cells, basophils have receptors for IgE antibodies, and crosslinking of these receptors can lead to basophil degranulation.

Although mast cells and basophils are responsible for the immediate reaction to an allergen, a third

granule-containing white blood cell, the **eosinophil**, is the prominent player in chronic allergic reactions (e.g., in asthma). Before an "attack" by an allergen, there are relatively few eosinophils present in the tissues or circulating in the blood. However, once an allergic reaction has begun, helper T cells secrete cytokines such as IL-5, which can recruit many more eosinophils from the bone marrow. These eosinophils can then add their "weight" to the allergic reaction. Because eosinophils must be mobilized from the marrow, their contribution is delayed relative to that of mast cells and basophils, which can respond almost immediately.

Of course, mast cells, basophils, and eosinophils were not invented by Mother Nature just to annoy atopic people. These cells, with their ability to degranulate "on command," provide a defense against parasites (e.g., worms) that are too large to be phagocytosed by professional phagocytes. In a sense, IgE antibodies act as a "guidance system" for these cells, targeting their weapons to the enemy. For example, by discharging their destructive chemicals directly onto the skin (tegument) of a parasite to which IgE antibodies have bound, eosinophils can destroy these massive creatures.

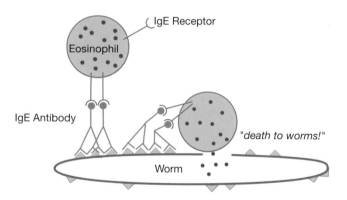

What makes this defense so elegant is that in response to a parasitic infection, parasite-specific IgE antibodies are made and mast cells, basophils, and eosinophils are armed. However, nothing happens unless these armed cells come in contact with a parasite that can cluster their IgE receptors. Consequently, you don't get uncontrolled degranulation, wreaking havoc throughout your body. Rather, the IgE guidance system allows these cells to zero in on parasites, causing relatively little collateral damage to our tissues.

Why do some people have allergies?

It is clear that IgE antibodies are the bad guys in allergic reactions, but what determines whether a person will make IgE or IgG antibodies in response to an allergen? You remember from Lecture 6 that helper T cells can be "instructed" by the environment in which they are stimulated to secrete various cytokine subsets (e.g., Th1, Th2, or Th17). And the cytokines given off by these T cells can then influence B cells undergoing class switching to produce IgA, IgG, or IgE antibodies. For example, a germinal center that is populated with Th1 cells usually will produce B cells that make IgG antibodies, because Th1 cells secrete IFN-γ, which drives the IgG class switch. In contrast, B cells tend to change to IgE production if class switching takes place in germinal centers that contain Th2 cells which secrete IL-4 and IL-5. Consequently, **the decision to produce either IgG or IgE antibodies in response to an allergen will depend heavily on the type of helper T cells present in the secondary lymphoid organ which happens to intercept the allergen.** Indeed, helper T cells from allergic individuals show a much stronger bias toward the Th2 type than do Th cells from non-atopic people.

The hygiene hypothesis

So atopic individuals produce IgE antibodies because their allergen-specific helper T cells tend to be of the Th2 type. But how do they get that way? The answer to this important question is not known for certain, but many immunologists believe that a bias toward Th2-type helper T cells can be established early in childhood, and in some cases, even before birth. Here's how this is thought to work.

A fetus inherits roughly half of its genetic material from its mother and half from its father. As a result, the fetus is really a "transplant" that expresses many paternal antigens to which the mother's immune system is not tolerant. Since the placenta is the interface between the mother and the fetus, measures must be taken to avoid having maternal CTLs and NK cells attack the placenta because it expresses these paternal antigens. The Th1 subset of helper cells secretes TNF, which helps activate NK cells, and IL-2, which causes NK cells and CTLs to proliferate. So it would be advantageous for the survival of the fetus to bias maternal Th cells away from the Th1 cytokine profile. Indeed, cells of the placenta produce relatively large amounts of IL-4, which influences maternal helper T cells to become Th2 cells. Importantly, these same placental cytokines also have a strong influence on <u>fetal</u> helper T cells. As a result, most humans are born with helper T cells that are strongly biased toward making Th2 cytokines.

Obviously this bias does not last a lifetime, and eventually most people end up with a more balanced population of Th1 and Th2 cells. One event that probably helps establish this balance is infection at an early age with microbes (e.g., viruses or bacteria) that normally elicit a Th1 response. Indeed, it is suspected that early microbial infections may be important in "reprogramming" a child's immune system so that a Th1 response to allergens results. Immunologists hypothesize that if a microbial infection strongly biases the immune response toward a Th1 type at the same time that the child encounters an allergen (say, a dust mite protein), the Th response to that allergen also will be deviated toward the Th1 type. Once this deviation takes place, feedback mechanisms tend to lock in the Th1 bias, and memory T cells will be generated that remember not only the allergen, but also their Th1 response to it. Once a large number of biased memory cells is built up, it is difficult to reverse this bias, so early exposure to infectious diseases may be critical in establishing a normal reaction to environmental allergens.

The idea that childhood microbial infections or early exposure to allergens might be important in biasing our immune systems toward producing Th1 helper T cells in response to environmental allergens is called the **hygiene hypothesis**. Indeed, in Western countries, where improved personal hygiene has led to a decrease in childhood infections, and where exposure to certain allergens early in life is less frequent, the incidence of allergies to environmental allergens has increased dramatically. Some of the best data in support of the hygiene hypothesis comes from studies of families living on traditional farms. These studies have shown that children who grow up on farms have a significantly lower incidence of asthma and hay fever than do children from rural areas who do not live on a farm. This effect is even more pronounced if their mothers come in contact with multiple animal species and animal feed (such as hay and grain) during their pregnancy. Interestingly, the timing of exposure to animals and their feed seems to be important, with the greatest protection being observed for children who live on a farm during the first few years of life. In this regard, it is important to note that living on a farm is not "unusual" as far as the human immune system is concerned. After all, until recently, many of our ancestors lived in close contact with farm animals, and it is likely that the immune system evolved to function best – at least in terms of allergies – in that setting.

In actual fact this probably should be called the "lifestyle hypothesis," because the increased incidence of allergies likely is due to a change in lifestyle, not just to improved hygiene or moving from a farm to the city. For example, prior to the 1950s, when televisions became commonplace in the United States, most children came home from school and went outdoors to play. Things are very different now, with many young children spending long hours indoors in front of the TV or the computer. Also, after World War II, it became customary for childhood illnesses to be treated with antibiotics, which can destroy intestinal bacteria that are helpful in setting up a "balanced" immune system. Indeed, studies show an increased risk of asthma in children who were treated with multiple courses of antibiotics during their first year of life.

It also has been proposed that regulatory T cells may help bias the immune system away from the production of IgE antibodies in response to environmental allergens. Helper T cells out in the tissues can be induced to become regulatory T cells (iTregs). Consequently, one could argue that if a person is routinely exposed to environmental allergens, some of his CD4$^+$ T cells may be induced to become regulatory T cells, which could suppress the immune response to these allergens. Indeed, inducible regulatory T cells produce IL-10 and TGFβ – cytokines which are known to bias antibody production away from IgE and toward IgG or IgA. Moreover, in individuals who are not atopic, regulatory T cells represent the majority of CD4$^+$ T cells that are specific for common environmental allergens. Although the idea that the induction of allergen-specific regulatory T cells might protect us from allergic reactions makes sense, more research is required to validate this hypothesis.

Heredity

In addition to environmental factors (e.g., early exposure to infectious diseases or environmental allergens), heredity clearly plays a large part in susceptibility to allergies. For example, if one identical twin suffers from allergies, the probability is about 50% that the second twin will also be atopic. Immunologists have noticed that people who are allergic to certain allergens are more likely to have inherited particular class II MHC genes than are non-atopic people, suggesting that these MHC molecules may be especially efficient at presenting allergens. Also, some atopic individuals produce mutant forms of the IgE receptor. It is hypothesized that these mutant receptors send an unusually strong signal when crosslinked, resulting in secretion of abnormally high levels of IL-4 by mast cells – which favor the production of IgE antibodies.

Likewise, in response to inflammation, thymic stromal lymphopoietin (TSLP) is produced by the epithelial cells that line the lungs. This cytokine can recruit and activate IL-4-producing immune cells, and certain mutations in the gene encoding TSLP are associated with an increased incidence of asthma. Unfortunately, mutations in genes that confer susceptibility to allergies have been difficult to identify because there seem to be many of them – and because they differ from atopic individual to atopic individual.

The best current synthesis of this information is that **the immunological basis for allergies is a defect in immune regulation in which allergen-specific helper T cells are strongly polarized toward a Th2 cytokine profile, resulting in the production of allergen-specific IgE antibodies. The genes a person inherits can make him more or less susceptible to allergies, and exposure to environmental factors such as microbial infections may influence whether susceptible individuals become atopic.**

It is important to recognize that allergies were not a major issue for our ancestors. They were not blessed with the good hygiene we have today, and were exposed at an early age to infectious diseases that most likely deviated their response to allergens away from the abnormal production of IgE antibodies. In fact, while many Americans may curse IgE antibodies, people in much of the rest of the world depend heavily on these antibodies to defend them against parasites. Indeed, parasitic worms infect roughly a third of the human population today.

Treatments for allergies

Although not a cure, treatment with glucocorticoid steroids can decrease allergy symptoms by blocking cytokine production by helper T cells. As a result, fewer B cells are activated (because they do not get the help they need), and the total number of antibodies made is reduced. Steroids, however, are not specific for allergies, and steroid treatment decreases the number of activated B cells of all kinds. Consequently, taking glucocorticoid steroids for extended periods can result in increased susceptibility to infectious diseases.

Recently, immunologists have produced antibodies (omalizumab) which can grasp the Fc region of IgE antibodies and block the binding of these antibodies to mast cells. In human trials, these blocking antibodies relieved allergic symptoms and decreased the severity of asthma attacks. This treatment has now been approved for use in the United States, and it appears to be safe and effective – especially in severe cases.

So far, only one approach, **specific immunotherapy**, has been successful in curing allergies. This treatment involves the injection of gradually increasing doses of crude extracts of allergens until a maintenance dose is achieved. Then, after several years of regular injections, some patients become tolerant to the allergen (or allergens) in the extract. Somehow, these injections encourage allergen-specific B cells to switch their antibody class from IgE to one of the other antibody classes. Indeed, during specific immunotherapy, the ratio of IgG to IgE antibodies specific for the allergen being administered can increase 10- to 100-fold. Unfortunately, the mechanism by which this immune deviation is achieved is not well understood. The latest thinking is that repeated injections of allergen extracts may generate inducible regulatory T cells which produce cytokines that suppress IgE antibody production. Interestingly, this view is supported by the finding that beekeepers, who receive repetitive doses of bee venom (because they are stung frequently), do not suffer severe allergic reactions when stung by bees, and have elevated levels of IL-10 – a cytokine produced by iTregs.

AUTOIMMUNE DISEASE

Rather than expend a huge amount of biological "energy" on a foolproof system in which every B and T cell is carefully checked for tolerance of self, Mother Nature evolved a multilayered system in which each layer includes mechanisms that should weed out most self-reactive cells, with lower layers catching cells that slip through tolerance induction in the layers above. This strategy works very well, but occasionally "mistakes are made" and instead of defending us against foreign invaders, the weapons of our immune system are turned back on us. **Autoimmune disease results when a breakdown in the mechanisms meant to preserve tolerance of self is severe enough to cause a pathological condition.** Roughly 5% of Americans suffer from some form of autoimmune disease.

Some cases of autoimmunity result from genetic defects. For example, most autoimmune diseases are chronic disorders that involve repeated stimulation of self-reactive lymphocytes. In healthy people, this is controlled by activation-induced cell death in which chronically stimulated T cells are eliminated when Fas proteins on their surface are ligated. Humans with genetic defects in either the Fas or the Fas ligand protein lack this layer of tolerance protection, and their T cells refuse to die when chronically stimulated by self antigens. The resulting disease, **autoimmune lymphoproliferative syndrome** or **Canale–Smith syndrome**, has, as its pathological consequences, massive swelling of lymph nodes, the production of antibodies that recognize self antigens, and the accumulation of a large number of T cells in the secondary lymphoid organs.

Although some autoimmune disorders are caused by genetic defects, **the majority of autoimmune diseases occur when the layers of tolerance-inducing mechanisms fail to eliminate self-reactive cells in genetically normal individuals.** In fact, you could argue that the potential for autoimmune disease is the price we must pay for having B and T cell receptors which are so diverse that they can recognize essentially any invader.

The latest thinking is that for autoimmunity to occur, at least three conditions must be met. First, an individual must express MHC molecules that efficiently present a peptide derived from the target self antigen. This means that the MHC molecules you inherit can play a major role in determining your susceptibility to autoimmune disease. For example, only about 0.2% of the U.S. population suffers from juvenile diabetes, yet for Caucasian Americans who inherit two particular types of class II MHC genes, the probability of contracting this autoimmune disease is increased about 20-fold.

The second requirement for autoimmunity is that the afflicted person must produce T and, in some cases, B cells which have receptors that recognize a self antigen. Because TCRs and BCRs are made by a mix-and-match strategy, the repertoire of receptors that one individual expresses will be different from that of every other human, and will change with time as lymphocytes die and are replaced. Even the collections of TCRs and BCRs expressed by identical twins will be different. Therefore, it is largely by chance that a person will produce lymphocytes whose receptors recognize a particular self antigen.

So for autoimmune disease to occur, a person must **have MHC molecules that can present a self antigen, and lymphocytes with receptors that can recognize the self antigen – but this is not enough. There also must be environmental factors that lead to the breakdown of the tolerance mechanisms which are designed to eliminate self-reactive lymphocytes.** For years, physicians have noticed that autoimmune diseases frequently follow bacterial or viral infections, and immunologists believe that microbial attack may be one of the key environmental factors that triggers autoimmune disease. Now clearly, a viral or bacterial infection cannot be the whole story, because for most people, these infections do not result in autoimmunity. However, in conjunction with a genetic predisposition (e.g., the type of MHC molecules inherited) and lymphocytes with potentially self-reactive receptors, a microbial infection may be the "last straw" that leads to autoimmune disease.

Molecular mimicry

Immunologists' current favorite hypothesis to explain why infections might lead to the breakdown of self tolerance is called **molecular mimicry**. Here's how this is thought to work.

Lymphocytes have BCRs or TCRs that recognize their cognate antigen. It turns out, however, that this is almost never a single antigen. Just as one MHC molecule can present a large number of peptides which have the same overall characteristics (length, binding motif, etc.), a TCR or a BCR usually can recognize (**cross react with**) several different antigens. Generally, a TCR or BCR will have a high affinity for one or a few of these cognate antigens, and relatively lower affinities for the others.

During a microbial invasion, lymphocytes whose receptors recognize microbial antigens will be activated. The molecular mimicry hypothesis holds that sometimes these receptors also recognize a self antigen, and if they do, an autoimmune response to that self antigen may result. It is presumed that before the microbial infection, these potentially self-reactive lymphocytes had not been activated – either because the affinity of their receptors for the self antigen was too low to trigger activation, or because the restricted traffic patterns of virgin lymphocytes never brought them into contact with the self antigen under conditions that would allow activation.

Another opportunity for generating self-reactive B cells may occur during somatic hypermutation. During this process, the receptors of a B cell that originally recognized only a bona fide pathogen could mutate so that they now recognize both the pathogen – making them "eligible" for Tfh help – and a self antigen – making them potentially destructive.

In these scenarios, the invading microbe substitutes for (mimics) the self antigen for activation. And once activated in response to a cross-reacting microbial antigen, these self-reactive lymphocytes can do real damage. Cross-reactive antibodies have been identified in some patients with autoimmune disease, and who previously had been infected by certain viruses or bacteria. For example, it is believed that **rheumatic heart disease**, which is a possible complication of a streptococcal throat infection, can result when receptors on helper T cells that recognize

streptococcal antigens cross react with a protein which is present on the tissues that make up the mitral valve of the heart. These cross-reactive Th cells appear to direct an inflammatory response that can severely damage this heart valve.

One reason it has been so difficult to pin down the environmental triggers for most autoimmune diseases is that TCRs which recognize self antigens usually can cross react with multiple environmental antigens. Consequently, **although viral or bacterial infections may be involved in some autoimmune disorders, it appears unlikely that any single microbe is responsible for any one autoimmune disease.**

Animal models of human autoimmune diseases have been useful for understanding which immune system players are involved, which self antigens are targets of the immune response, and which microbial antigens might be involved in the molecular mimicry that may trigger disease. Typically, these models involve animals that have been bred to be exquisitely susceptible to autoimmune disease, or animals whose genes have been altered to make them susceptible. Nevertheless, animal models frequently differ in important respects from the human disease they are meant to model. As a result, many treatments for autoimmune diseases which look promising in an animal model have turned out to be useless in humans.

Inflammation and autoimmune disease

Although molecular mimicry may result in the activation of lymphocytes that previously had been ignorant of self antigens, these self-reactive lymphocytes still face a problem once they reach the tissues where the self antigen is located: They must be reactivated before they can do any real damage. If the innate immune system is battling an infection in the tissues, inflammatory cytokines such as IFN-γ and TNF secreted by cells of the innate system will activate APCs (e.g., macrophages) that reside in the tissues. Once activated, these APCs express the MHC and co-stimulatory molecules required to re-stimulate T cells which enter the tissues to do battle. Consequently, when lymphocytes venture out into the tissues to join a war that the innate system is already fighting, re-stimulation is not a problem. However, for a T cell that recognizes a self antigen which the innate system does not see as dangerous, the tissues can be a very inhospitable place – because that self-reactive lymphocyte usually will not receive the co-stimulation necessary for its survival.

What this means is that it is not enough for a microbe to activate self-reactive T cells by mimicry. There also must be an inflammatory reaction going on in the same tissues that express the self antigen. Otherwise it is unlikely that self-reactive lymphocytes would exit the blood into these tissues, and, if they did, that they would survive. This requirement for inflammation at the site of an autoimmune attack helps explains why, for example, a strep infection in the throat only rarely leads to rheumatic heart disease.

So the scenario most immunologists favor for the initiation of autoimmune disease is this: **A genetically susceptible individual is attacked by a microbe that activates T cells whose receptors just happen to cross react with a self antigen. Simultaneously, an inflammatory reaction takes place in the tissues where the self antigen is expressed. This inflammation could be caused either by the mimicking microbe itself, or by another, unrelated infection or trauma. As a result of this inflammatory reaction, APCs are activated that can re-stimulate self-reactive T cells. In addition, cytokines generated by the inflammatory response can upregulate class I MHC expression on normal cells in the tissues, making these cells even better targets for destruction by self-reactive CTLs.**

Examples of autoimmune disease

Autoimmune diseases usually are divided into two groups: organ-specific and systemic diseases. Let's look at examples of both types, paying special attention to the self antigens against which the autoimmune response is thought to be directed, and to the environmental antigens that may be involved in molecular mimicry.

Insulin-dependent diabetes mellitus (type 1 diabetes) is an example of an organ-specific autoimmune disease. In this disease, the targets of autoimmune attack are the insulin-producing β cells of the pancreas. Although antibodies produced by self-reactive B cells may participate in the chronic inflammation that contributes to the pathology of this disease, it is currently believed that the initial attack on the β cells is mediated by CTLs.

Clearly, there are genetic factors that help determine susceptibility to diabetes, since the probability that both identical twins will suffer from this autoimmune disease is about 50% if one of them has it. It is known, for example, that some individuals have a version of the gene for CTLA-4 which is associated with an increased risk of type 1 diabetes. Patients with this variant make less CTLA-4 RNA, and presumably are less able to limit the activity of self-reactive T cells that recognize β cell antigens.

Thus far, no strong candidates have emerged for environmental factors that might trigger the initial attack on β cells. However, many immunologists believe that diabetes results, at least in part, when the balance between natural regulatory T cells and potentially self-reactive CTLs is upset. Indeed, mutations in genes that compromise nTreg function can cause autoimmune disease both in humans and in mice.

In diabetes, destruction of insulin-producing cells in the pancreas usually begins months or even years before the first symptoms of diabetes appear, so this disease is sometimes referred to as a "silent killer." Indeed, by the time symptoms appear, more than 90% of a patient's β cells usually will have been destroyed. Fortunately, antibodies that bind to β cell antigens are produced very early in the disease. As a result, relatives of diabetic patients can be tested to determine whether they might be in the initial stages of diabetes, and could be helped by early intervention. Indeed, if a child has a sibling who developed diabetes early in life, and if that child's immune system does make antibodies which recognize beta cell proteins, the probability that he will develop diabetes within the next five years is nearly 100%.

Myasthenia gravis is an autoimmune disease that results when self-reactive antibodies bind to the receptor for an important neurotransmitter, acetylcholine. When the message that is normally carried by acetylcholine from nerve to muscle is not received (because the antibodies interfere with its reception), muscle weakness and paralysis can result. Immunologists have noticed that a region of one of the poliovirus proteins is similar in amino acid sequence to part of the acetylcholine receptor protein, so it is possible that a polio infection might provide one mimic which could activate lymphocytes whose receptors cross react with the acetylcholine receptor.

Multiple sclerosis is an inflammatory disease of the central nervous system that is thought to be initiated by self-reactive T cells. In multiple sclerosis, chronic inflammation destroys the myelin sheaths that are required for nerve cells in the brain to transmit electrical signals efficiently, causing defects in sensory inputs (e.g., vision) and paralysis. Macrophages recruited by cytokines secreted by T cells are thought to play a major role in causing this inflammation. At first there was a question as to how T cells could get into the brain to initiate this disease, but eventually it was discovered that activated T cells (but not virgin T cells) can cross the blood–brain barrier. The presumed target of these T cells is a major component of the myelin sheath: **myelin basic protein**. T cells isolated from multiple sclerosis patients can recognize a peptide derived from myelin basic protein as well as peptides derived from proteins encoded by both herpes simplex virus and Epstein–Barr virus (the virus that causes mononucleosis). So a possible scenario is that when genetically susceptible individuals are infected with herpes virus or Epstein–Barr virus, they produce T cells that recognize proteins from these viruses. Some of these activated T cells may have receptors that cross react with myelin basic protein, and once these T cells cross the blood–brain barrier, they can lead the attack on the myelin sheaths, causing the symptoms of multiple sclerosis.

Of course, very few people who have Epstein–Barr or herpes infections get multiple sclerosis, so exposure to microbial mimics is not the whole story. Indeed, as is true of most autoimmune diseases, multiple sclerosis has a strong genetic component: It is about 10 times more probable that identical twins will share this disease than it is for non-identical twins both to be afflicted. In addition, it is about 20 times more likely that the non-identical twin of someone with multiple sclerosis also will have the disease than it is for a person in the general population. There also are certain "resistant" groups (e.g., Hispanic, Asian, and Native American) who have relatively low rates of multiple sclerosis, presumably because of their particular genetic makeup. Nevertheless, the only gene that has been shown conclusively to confer increased susceptibility to multiple sclerosis is a particular class II MHC gene.

Rheumatoid arthritis is a systemic autoimmune disease that affects approximately 1% of the world's population. It is characterized by chronic inflammation of the joints. One of the presumed targets of this autoimmune reaction is a certain cartilage protein, and T cells from arthritic patients can recognize both the cartilage protein and a protein encoded by the bacterium that causes tuberculosis. Moreover, mice injected with *Mycobacterium tuberculosis* develop inflammation of the joints, suggesting, but not proving, that a mycobacterial infection may trigger rheumatoid arthritis in some patients.

IgM antibodies that can bind to the Fc region of IgG antibodies are abundant in the joints of individuals with rheumatoid arthritis. These antibodies can form IgM–IgG antibody complexes, which can activate macrophages that have entered the joints, increasing the inflammatory reaction. Indeed, the inflammation associated with rheumatoid arthritis is caused mainly by tumor necrosis factor produced by macrophages that infiltrate the joints under the direction of self-reactive helper T cells. To treat arthritis, several drugs are currently being used which "soak up" TNF. One type is an antibody that binds to TNF and prevents it from working, while another is a fake receptor for TNF. Both of these "blockade" strategies are very effective in decreasing the severity of the symptoms experienced by patients with rheumatoid arthritis.

Finally, **lupus erythematosus** is a systemic autoimmune disease that affects about 250 000 people in the United States, roughly 90% of whom are women. This disease can have multiple manifestations including a red rash on the forehead and cheeks (giving the "red wolf" appearance for which the disease was named), inflammation of the lungs, arthritis, kidney damage, hair loss, paralysis, and convulsions. Lupus is caused by a breakdown in both B and T cell tolerance that results in the production of a diverse collection of IgG antibodies which recognize a wide range of self antigens, including DNA, DNA–protein complexes, and RNA–protein complexes. These autoantibodies can form self antigen–antibody complexes which "clog" organs in the body that contain "filters" (e.g., kidneys, joints, and the brain), causing chronic inflammation.

Non-identical twins have about a 2% probability of both having lupus if one twin has the disease. With identical twins, the probability is increased about 10-fold. This indicates a strong genetic component to the disease, and more than a dozen MHC and non-MHC genes have been identified – each of which seems to slightly increase the probability that a person will contract lupus. Although no specific microbial infection has been associated with the initiation of this autoimmune disease, mice that lack functional genes for Fas or Fas ligand exhibit lupus-like symptoms. This has led immunologists to speculate that lupus may involve a defect in activation-induced cell death, in which lymphocytes that should die due to chronic stimulation survive to cause the disease. There is also some evidence that humans with mutations which increase the sensitivity of their Toll-like receptors to RNA or DNA are lupus-prone. The idea here is that recognition of human DNA by a B cell's receptors, together with an unusually strong signal from a mutated Toll-like receptor, could be misinterpreted as a dangerous situation. As a result, B cells could be activated without T cell help, and anti-DNA antibodies could be produced.

REVIEW

Most of the time, the immune system functions flawlessly, but occasionally it "makes mistakes." Some of these mistakes are the result of special situations in which the system functions as designed, but the response actually contributes to the disease. In other cases, the immune response may be misguided. Indeed, allergies result when the immune system produces IgE antibodies – which are designed to deal with a parasitic infection – in response to environmental antigens. Immunologists are not sure what causes this misguided response. Their best thought is that a defect in immune regulation causes production of a large number of allergen-specific Th2 cells. These helper T cells then orchestrate the overproduction of allergen-specific IgE antibodies. Atopic individuals frequently inherit a "genetic landscape" which predisposes them to allergies, and the timing and extent of exposure to pathogens may influence whether susceptible individuals become atopic. In fact, the hygiene hypothesis holds that if the immune system of a child is not appropriately challenged by microbial infections, allergies can result.

Autoimmunity results when the mechanisms designed to enforce tolerance of self antigens don't function properly. In some cases, this is the result of genetic defects. However, in most cases, immunologists don't know what causes the breakdown in tolerance-inducing mechanisms. Clearly, for autoimmunity to occur, a person must have MHC molecules which can present self antigens, and lymphocytes with receptors that can recognize these antigens. So there is a genetic component. In addition, it is believed that environmental factors are involved, although such factors have been difficult to discover – probably because there are many of them. The current best hypothesis is that autoimmunity can be triggered when an invading microbe "mimics" a self antigen. According to this scenario, the microbe activates lymphocytes which have receptors that recognize both a microbial antigen and a self antigen. Once activated in response to the microbial invasion, these cross-reactive lymphocytes can lead an attack on both the invader and the cells or proteins belonging to the infected individual. Inflammation also is believed to play a role in autoimmunity by helping reactivate cross-reactive lymphocytes.

THOUGHT QUESTIONS

1. Describe the events that lead to the degranulation of mast cells during an allergic reaction.

2. Why do some people have allergies, whereas others do not?

3. What events likely are required to initiate autoimmunity?

LECTURE 14 Immunodeficiency

HEADS UP!

Because the immune system is highly interconnected, a genetic defect which cripples one of the players can have a major effect on the functioning of the overall system. Moreover, drugs or illnesses which weaken the immune system can leave us vulnerable to infections – infections which would not be a problem for an immune system operating at full strength.

INTRODUCTION

Serious disease may result when our immune system is compromised. Some immunodeficiencies are caused by genetic defects that disable parts of the immune network. Others are "acquired" as the consequence of malnutrition, deliberate immunosuppression (e.g., during organ transplantation or chemotherapy for cancer), or disease (e.g., AIDS).

GENETIC DEFECTS LEADING TO IMMUNODEFICIENCY

A genetic defect in which a single gene is mutated can lead to immune system weakness. For example, individuals who are born with non-functional CD40 or CD40L proteins are unable to mount a T cell-dependent antibody response because T cells either cannot deliver or B cells cannot receive this all-important,

co-stimulatory signal. Both class switching and somatic hypermutation usually require co-stimulation by CD40L, so one result of the CD40–CD40L defect is that B cells secrete mainly IgM antibodies which have not affinity matured. Other genetic deficiencies affect the formation of the thymus. In one such disease, DiGeorge syndrome, essentially all thymic tissue is missing. People with this disorder are susceptible to life-threatening infections because they lack functional T cells.

Genetic defects also can knock out both B and T cells. This group of diseases is called **severe combined immunodeficiency syndrome (SCIDS)** – where the "combined" label indicates that neither B nor T cells function properly. It was this disease that forced David Vetter, the famous "bubble boy," to live for 12 years in a pathogen-free plastic bubble. Although a number of different mutations can result in SCIDS, the best-studied mutation causes a defect in a protein that initiates the gene splicing required to produce B and T cell receptors. Without their receptors, B and T cells are totally useless.

Immunodeficiencies also can result from genetic defects in the innate immune system. For example, people who are born with mutations in important complement proteins such as C3 have lymph nodes with an abnormal architecture (no germinal centers) and B cells which produce mainly IgM antibodies.

Given the large number of different proteins involved in making the innate and adaptive immune systems work effectively, it's pretty amazing that mutations leading to immunodeficiency are so rare. In fact, inherited immunodeficiencies affect only about 1 in 10 000 newborns. It is likely, however, that many other cases of genetic immunodeficiency go undetected because our functionally redundant immune system has evolved to provide "backups" when elements of the main system are disabled.

AIDS

Although genetic immunodeficiencies are relatively rare, millions of people suffer from immunodeficiencies that are acquired. A large group of immunodeficient humans acquired their deficiency when they were infected with the AIDS virus – a virus that has infected at least 70 million people worldwide, resulting in more than 30 million deaths. The AIDS symptoms which originally alerted physicians that they were dealing with a disease which had immunodeficiency as its basis were the high incidence of infections (e.g., *Pneumocystis carinii* pneumonia) or cancers (e.g., Kaposi sarcoma) that usually were seen only in immunosuppressed individuals. Soon, the virus that caused this immunodeficiency was isolated and named the **human immunodeficiency virus number one (HIV-1)**. Currently, this is the world's most intensely studied virus, with nearly a billion dollars being spent annually to try to discover its secrets.

An HIV-1 infection

The early events in a human HIV-1 infection are not well characterized because the infection typically is not diagnosed until weeks or months after exposure to the virus. However, the emerging picture is that these infections typically begin when the virus penetrates the rectal or vaginal mucosa and infects helper T cells which lie below these protective surfaces. The virus uses these cells' biosynthetic machinery to make many more copies of itself, and the newly made viruses then infect other cells. So in the early stages of infection, the virus multiplies relatively unchecked while the innate system gives it its best shot, and the adaptive system is being mobilized. After a week or so, the adaptive system starts to kick in, and virus-specific B cells, helper T cells, and CTLs are activated, proliferate, and begin to do their thing. During this early, **acute phase** of the infection, there is a dramatic rise in the number of viruses in the body (the **viral load**) as the virus multiplies in infected cells. The viral load peaks 3–4 weeks post infection, and this peak is followed by a marked decrease in the viral load as virus-specific CTLs go to work.

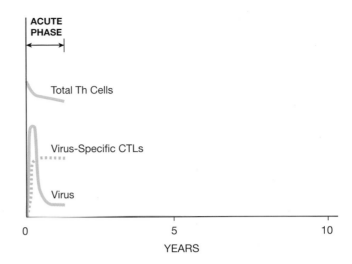

With many viruses (e.g., smallpox), the end result of the acute phase of a viral infection is **sterilization**: The immune system destroys all the invading viruses, and memory B and T cells are produced to protect against a subsequent infection by the same virus. In contrast, a full-blown HIV-1 infection always leads to a **chronic phase** that can last for 10 or more years. During this phase, a fierce struggle goes on between the immune system and the AIDS virus – a struggle which the virus almost always wins.

During the chronic phase of infection, viral loads decrease to low levels compared with those reached during the height of the acute phase, but the number of virus-specific CTLs and Th cells remains high – a sign that the immune system is still trying hard to defeat the virus.

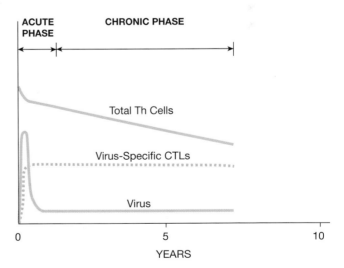

However, as the chronic phase progresses, the total number of helper T cells slowly decreases, because these cells are killed as a consequence of the viral infection. Eventually there are not enough Th cells left to provide the help needed by virus-specific CTLs. When this happens, the number of CTLs also begins to decline, and the viral load increases – because there are too few CTLs left to cope with newly infected cells.

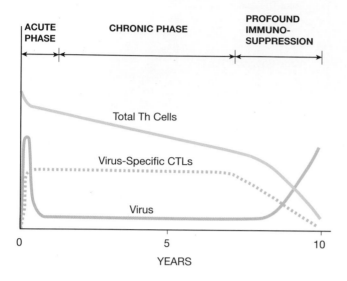

In the end, the immune defenses are overwhelmed, and the resulting profound state of immunosuppression leaves the patient open to unchecked infections by pathogens that normally would not be the slightest problem for a person with an intact immune system. Sadly, these **opportunistic infections** can be lethal to an AIDS patient whose immune system has been destroyed.

HIV-1 versus the immune system

Why is HIV-1 able to defeat an immune system that is so successful in protecting us from most other pathogens? There are two parts to this answer. The first has to do with the nature of the virus itself. All viruses are basically pieces of genetic information (either DNA or RNA) with a protective coat. For the AIDS virus, this genetic information is in the form of RNA which, after the virus enters its target cell, is copied by a viral enzyme (reverse transcriptase) to make a piece of "complementary" DNA (cDNA). Next, the DNA of the cell is cut by another enzyme carried by the virus, and the viral cDNA is inserted into the gap in the cellular DNA. Now comes the nasty part. Once the viral DNA has been inserted into a cell's DNA, it can just sit there, and while the virus is in this "latent" state, the infected cell cannot be detected by CTLs. Recent data suggests that it takes only 5–10 days for HIV-1 to initiate a **latent infection** and establish a **stealth reservoir of virus** in these "sanctuary" cells. Some time later, in response to signals that are not fully understood, the latent virus can be "reactivated,"

additional copies of the virus can be produced, and more cells can be infected by these newly minted viruses.

The fact that a reservoir of virus which is "invisible" to the immune system can be established within a week or so of infection is a serious problem. After all, a week into the infection, the adaptive immune system is still being activated. Consequently, the major responsibility for stopping the virus before it can get a "foothold" falls to the innate system. And the innate immune system usually is not up to the task.

So **the ability to quickly establish a latent infection which cannot be detected by CTLs is one property of HIV-1 that makes this virus such a problem for the immune system.** But it gets worse. The reverse transcriptase enzyme used to copy the HIV-1 RNA is very error-prone: It makes a "mistake" almost every time it copies a piece of viral RNA. This means that most of the new viruses produced by an infected cell are mutated versions of the virus which originally infected that cell. And some of these mutations may enable the newly made viruses to evade the immune system. For example, the virus can mutate so that a viral peptide that formerly was targeted by a CTL no longer can be recognized, or no longer can be presented by the MHC molecule that the CTL was trained to focus on. In fact, it has been shown that it only takes about 10 days for these **escape mutants** to arise. When such mutations occur, the original CTL will be useless against cells infected with the mutant virus, and new CTLs which recognize another viral peptide will need to be activated. Meanwhile, the virus that has escaped from surveillance by the obsolete CTLs is replicating like crazy, and every time it infects a new cell, it mutates again. Consequently, the mutation rate of the AIDS virus is so high that it usually can stay one step ahead of CTLs or antibodies directed against it.

So two of the properties of HIV-1 that make it especially deadly are its ability to establish an undetectable, latent infection, and its high mutation rate. But that's only half the story. The other part has to do with the cells HIV-1 infects. This virus specifically targets cells of the immune system: helper T cells, macrophages, and dendritic cells. The "docking" protein that HIV-1 binds to when it infects a cell is CD4, the co-receptor protein found in large numbers on the surface of helper T cells. This protein also is expressed on macrophages and dendritic cells, although they have fewer CD4 molecules on their surface. By attacking these cells, the AIDS virus either disrupts their function, kills the cells, or makes them targets for killing by CTLs that recognize them as being virus-infected. So the very cells that are needed to activate CTLs and to provide them with help are damaged or destroyed by the virus.

Even more insidiously, **HIV-1 can turn the immune system against itself by using processes which are essential for immune function to spread and maintain the viral infection.** For example, HIV-1 can attach to the surface of dendritic cells and be transported by these cells from the tissues, where there are relatively few CD4+ cells, into the lymph nodes, where huge numbers of CD4+ T cells are located. Not only are helper T cells within easy reach in the lymph nodes, but many of these cells are proliferating, making them ideal candidates to be infected and become HIV-1 "factories."

Also, AIDS viruses that have been opsonized either by antibodies or by complement are retained in lymph nodes by follicular dendritic cells. This display is intended to help activate B cells. However, CD4+ T cells also pass through these forests of follicular dendritic cells, and as they do, they can be infected by the opsonized AIDS viruses. And because virus particles typically remain bound to follicular dendritic cells for months, lymph nodes actually become reservoirs of HIV-1. The net result is that HIV-1 takes advantage of the normal trafficking of immune system cells through lymph nodes, and turns these secondary lymphoid organs into its own playground.

In summary, **the pathological consequences of an HIV-1 infection are the result of the virus' ability to slowly destroy the immune system of the patient, leading to a state of profound immunosuppression which makes the individual an inviting host for life-threatening infections. The virus is able to do this because it can rapidly establish a latent, "stealth" infection, because it has a high mutation rate, because it preferentially infects and disables the immune system cells that normally would defend against it, and because it uses the immune system itself to facilitate its spread throughout the body.**

Living with AIDS

Untreated, most people infected with HIV-1 die within 10 years. Fortunately, for those who can afford it, chemotherapy (**h**ighly **a**ctive **a**nti-**r**etroviral **t**reatment) is now available which targets specific aspects of the viral replication cycle, and can lengthen the life of an AIDS patient by many years. However, **HAART** is not without side effects. Indeed, for those on HAART, there is an increased risk for cancer and cognitive disorders, as well as kidney, liver, bone, and heart disease. As a result, the average life span of a person on HAART is about 20 years less than that of a person who has not been infected with HIV-1.

Interestingly, for a very small fraction of untreated individuals infected with HIV-1 (roughly 0.3%), their immune system is able to control the infection for a relatively long period of time. In fact, some of these **elite controllers** have almost undetectable levels of virus, and have remained symptom-free for as long as 30 years. As you might expect, immunologists are very interested in understanding how the immune system of an elite controller deals with a viral infection that is deadly for most other humans. Although the story is far from complete, there are some clues.

One consistent finding is that innate and adaptive defenses of elite controllers seem to fire up more quickly after the initial infection than does the immune system of "ordinary" humans. Several possible reasons for this quick response have been discovered. For example, the pattern-recognition receptors of some elite controllers trigger unusually vigorous secretion of IFN-α and IFN-β by cells of the innate immune system. These "warning cytokines" cause infected cells to die by apoptosis, destroying the viruses that are replicating inside them. In addition, IFN-α and IFN-β activate genes within infected cells that encode proteins which limit the efficiency of replication of the AIDS virus.

In Lecture 4, I noted that one reason MHC molecules are so polymorphic is to increase the probability that at least some individuals in the population will have MHC molecules that can bind to and present an invader's peptides. This idea is supported by the finding that certain class I MHC molecules are found much more often in elite controllers than in the general population. The thinking here is that because these MHC molecules efficiently present HIV-1 peptides, killer T cells will be activated earlier in an infection when the number of infected cells is still small. In addition, when CTLs from elite controllers are tested in the laboratory, they tend to be more vicious killers than CTLs from patients who cannot control the infection. This seems to be due to the ability of these "super CTLs" to mobilize the killing enzyme granzyme B, and to deliver it into its target cells. Again, the thinking is that these CTLs kill faster, and can control the infection before it gets out of hand.

Of course, the hope is that if the unique features of the immune system of elite controllers can be understood in more detail, this information may be helpful in devising new treatments for persons infected with HIV-1. It is important to understand, however, that elite controllers are still infected: They continue to have reservoirs of latently infected CD4+ T cells. Their immune system has not defeated the virus. It has only controlled it for an extended period of time.

So far, there is only one documented case of an AIDS patient who appears to have been treated and cured of the disease: the so-called "Berlin patient." After he was infected with HIV-1, this individual developed acute myelogenous leukemia. As treatment for that disease, he twice had his immune system destroyed by chemicals or radiation and reconstituted with stem cell transplants. The stem cell donor in both procedures had deletions in his genes for CCR5, the most common co-receptor for the AIDS virus. As of this writing, the Berlin patient is still free of cancer and HIV-1.

REVIEW

Mutations that are inherited or that arise spontaneously can cause the immune system to function suboptimally. Indeed about 1 in 10 000 newborns suffer from some form of "genetic" immunodeficiency. Other immunodeficiencies arise when the immune system is suppressed by drugs or disease.

Today, millions of humans are immunodeficient as a result of infection with the AIDS virus. HIV-1 goes at the immune system "head on" by infecting and destroying the very immune warriors which might otherwise defend against the attack. The virus uses the immune system to facilitate its spread throughout the body, and it can establish a "hidden" reservoir of virus within the immune system cells of an infected individual. In addition, because the virus mutates rapidly, killer T cells, which can recognize and kill infected cells, quickly become "obsolete," allowing the virus to stay one step ahead of the immune defenses.

Highly active anti-retroviral treatment, a form of chemotherapy, can be used to extend the life span of patients infected with HIV-1. However, these treatments are expensive and can have serious side effects. Untreated, most AIDS patients succumb to infections which the immune system of a healthy individual could easily defeat. Some "elite controllers" are chronically infected with the virus, but remain asymptomatic for long periods of time. Immunologists are eagerly examining the immune system of these "lucky few" to try to determine why they are able to control an infection which is lethal to so many others.

THOUGHT QUESTIONS

1. Describe what happens to a patient's immune system during the course of an HIV-1 infection.

2. Discuss the features of an HIV-1 infection that make it so difficult for the immune system to deal with.

3. In the past, when the human immune system has been confronted with new dangers, it has evolved to meet these challenges. Given enough time, what evolutionary changes would you predict that our immune system might make to defend us against HIV-1?

LECTURE 15 # Cancer and the Immune System

INTRODUCTION

In this lecture, we are going to discuss how the immune system deals with cancer. This is a disease that will touch us all, either directly or indirectly. Because you may not have had a cancer course, I will begin by discussing some general properties of cancer cells. After all, it's important to know the enemy.

CANCER IS A CONTROL SYSTEM PROBLEM

Cancer arises when multiple control systems within a single cell are corrupted. These control systems are of two basic types: systems that promote cell growth (proliferation), and safeguard systems that protect against "irresponsible" cell growth. When controlled properly, cell proliferation is a good thing. After all, an adult human is made up of trillions of cells, so a lot of proliferation must take place between the time we are a single, fertilized egg and the time we are full-grown. However, once a human reaches adulthood, most cell proliferation ceases. For example, when the cells in your kidney have proliferated to make that organ exactly the right size, kidney cells stop proliferating. On the other hand, skin cells and cells that line our body cavities

(e.g., our intestines) must proliferate almost continuously to replenish cells that are lost as these surfaces are eroded by normal wear and tear. All this cell proliferation, from cradle to grave, must be carefully controlled to insure that the right amount of proliferation occurs at the right places in the body – and at the right times.

Usually, the growth-promoting systems within our cells work just fine. However, occasionally one of these systems may malfunction, and a cell may begin to proliferate inappropriately. When this happens, that cell has taken the first step toward becoming a cancer cell. Because these growth-promoting systems are made up of proteins, malfunctions occur when gene expression is altered, usually as a result of a mutation. **A gene that, when mutated, can cause a cell to proliferate inappropriately is called a proto-oncogene. And the mutated version of such a gene is called an oncogene.** The important point here is that **uncontrolled cell growth can result when a normal cellular gene is mutated.**

To protect against malfunctions in the control systems that promote cell proliferation, Mother Nature has equipped cells with <u>internal</u> safeguard systems. These safeguards are of two general types: systems that help prevent mutations and systems that deal with these mutations once they occur. For example, cells have a number of different repair systems that can fix damaged DNA, helping safeguard against mutations. These DNA repair systems are especially important, because mutations occur continuously in the DNA of all our cells. In fact, it is estimated that, on average, each of our cells suffers about 25 000 mutational events every day. Fortunately, repair systems work non-stop, and if the DNA damage is relatively small, it can be repaired immediately as part of the "maintenance" repair program.

Sometimes, however, the maintenance repair systems may miss a mutation, especially when there are many mutations and the repair systems are overwhelmed. When this happens, a second type of safeguard system comes into play – one that monitors unrepaired mutations. If the mutations are not extensive, this safeguard system stops the cell from proliferating to give the repair systems more time to do their thing. However, if the genetic damage is severe, the safeguard system will trigger the cell to commit suicide, eliminating the possibility that it will become a cancer cell. One of the important components of this safeguard system is a protein called **p53**. **Proteins like p53, which help safeguard against uncontrolled cell growth, are called tumor suppressors, and the genes that encode them are called anti-oncogenes or tumor suppressor genes.** Mutations in p53 have been detected in the majority of human tumors, and scientists have created mice with mutant p53 genes. In contrast to normal mice, which rarely get cancer, mice that lack functional p53 proteins usually die of cancer before they are seven months old. So, if you are ever asked to give up one gene, don't pick p53!

The take-home lesson is that every normal cell has both proto-oncogenes and tumor suppressor genes. Where things get dangerous is when proto-oncogenes are mutated, so that the cell proliferates inappropriately, and tumor suppressor genes are mutated so that the cell can't defend itself against proto-oncogenes "gone wrong." Indeed, **cancer results when multiple control systems, both growth-promoting and safeguard, are corrupted within a single cell.** It is estimated that between four and seven such mutations are required to produce most common cancers. This is the reason why cancer is a disease which generally strikes late in life: It usually takes a long time to accumulate the multiple mutations required to inappropriately activate growth-promoting systems and to disable safeguard systems.

Mutations that affect growth-promoting systems and safeguard systems can occur in any order. However, one type of mutation that is especially insidious is a genetic alteration which disrupts a safeguard system involved in repairing mutated DNA. When this happens, the mutation rate in a cell can soar, making it much more likely that the cell will accrue the multiple mutations required to turn it into a cancer cell. This type of "mutation-accelerating" defect is found in many (perhaps all) cancer cells. Indeed, **one of the hallmarks of a cancer cell is a genetically unstable condition in which cellular genes are constantly mutating.**

CLASSIFICATION OF CANCER CELLS

Cancer cells can be grouped into two general categories: **non-blood cell cancers (usually referred to as solid tumors) and blood cell cancers. Solid tumors are further classified according to the cell type from which they arise. Carcinomas,** the most common tumors in humans, are cancers of epithelial cells, and include lung, breast, colon, and cervical cancer. These cancers generally kill by metastasizing to a vital organ, where they grow and crowd the organ until it no longer can function properly. Humans also get cancers of the connective and structural tissues, although these **sarcomas** are relatively rare compared to carcinomas. Perhaps the best known example of a sarcoma is bone cancer (osteosarcoma).

Blood cell cancers make up the other class of human cancers, and the most frequent of these are leukemias and lymphomas. Blood cell cancers arise when descendants of blood stem cells, which normally should mature into lymphocytes or myeloid cells (e.g., neutrophils) stop maturing, and just continue proliferating. In a real sense, these blood cells refuse to "grow up" – and that's the problem. In leukemia, the immature cells fill up the bone marrow and prevent other blood cells from maturing. As a result, the patient usually dies from anemia (due to a scarcity of red blood cells) or from infections (due to a deficit of immune system cells). In lymphoma, large "clusters" of immature cells form in lymph nodes and other secondary lymphoid organs – clusters that in some ways resemble solid tumors. Lymphoma patients usually succumb to infections or organ malfunction.

There is another way to classify human cancers: **spontaneous** and **virus-associated. Most human tumors are called spontaneous because they arise when a single cell accumulates a collection of mutations that causes it to acquire the properties of a cancer cell.** These mutations can result from errors made when cellular DNA is copied to be passed down to daughter cells, or from the effects of mutagenic compounds (**carcinogens**) that are byproducts of normal cellular metabolism – or that are present in the air we breathe and the food we eat. Mutations can also be caused by radiation (including UV light) or by errors made in assembling the segments of DNA that make up the B and T cell receptors. As we go through life, these mutations occur "spontaneously," but there are certain factors that can <u>accelerate</u> the rate of mutation: cigarette smoking, a fatty diet, an increased radiation exposure from living at high altitude, working in a pluto-nium processing plant, and so on.

In addition to mutations in cellular genes that can corrupt growth-promoting and safeguard systems, some viruses produce proteins that can interfere with the proper functioning of these same systems in virus-infected cells. Virus-associated cancers also are "spon-taneous" in the sense that mutations are involved. However, virus-associated cancers have, as an addi-tional accelerating factor, a viral infection. For example, essentially all human cervical cancers involve an infec-tion by the human papillomavirus. This sexually trans-mitted virus infects cells that line the uterine cervix, and expresses in these cells viral proteins that can disable two safeguard systems, including the p53 system. Likewise, hepatitis B virus can establish a chronic infection of liver cells, can inactivate p53, and can act as an accelerating factor for liver cancer. So the net effect of an infection with these special **tumor viruses** is to decrease the total number of cellular genes that must be mutated to turn a normal cell into a cancer cell.

The hallmark of virus-associated cancer is that only a small fraction of infected individuals actually get cancer, yet for those who do, virus or viral genes usually can be recovered from their tumors. For example, less than 1% of women infected with genital human papillomavirus will ever get cancer of the cervix, yet human papilloma-virus genes have been found in over 90% of all cervical carcinomas examined. The reason for this, of course, is that the virus can't cause cancer by itself – it can only accelerate the process that involves the accumulation of cancer-causing mutations. About one fifth of all human cancers have a viral infection as an accelerating factor.

IMMUNE SURVEILLANCE AGAINST CANCER

From this introduction, it should be clear that powerful defenses exist within the cell (e.g., tumor suppressor proteins) to deal harshly with most wannabe cancer cells. Whether or not the immune system also plays a major role in protecting us against the majority of human cancers is not nearly so clear.

In mice that have been engineered so that one or more of the components of their immune system is defective an increased incidence of lymphoma, leukemia, and virus-associated cancer is well documented. However, the evidence that mice with compromised immune sys-tems experience an increase in solid tumors that do not involve a virus infection is not compelling. Moreover, because there are significant differences between mouse and human immune systems, it is difficult to know which experiments with mice are relevant to human cancer. Indeed, about 90% of the anti-cancer drugs which show promise in mouse models fail in human trials.

If the immune system provides surveillance against precancerous cells and destroys them before they can form tumors, one would predict that humans with genetic defects that weaken their immune system would have a higher incidence of cancer than those whose immune system is functioning normally. This turns out to be the case. However, a close inspection of these stud-ies reveals that the increased cancer rate in these people is most likely due to an increased susceptibility to can-cer rather than a defect in immune surveillance against the cancer. For example, most human cancers caused by defective immune system genes are lymphomas or leuke-mias. The cause of these cancers can be traced to defects in B or T cell maturation, not to defective surveillance. Other cancers that arise in people with inherited genetic defects result from the inability of a weakened immune system to defend against cancer-associated viruses (i.e., not against the cancer itself) or against pathogens which cause chronic inflammation – which can predispose to cancer.

There is evidence that humans who are chemically immunosuppressed to avoid rejection of a transplanted organ do have higher than normal cancer rates. However, in these studies, it is possible that the immunosuppres-sive drugs increased the cancer incidence either directly, or indirectly by weakening the immune response against pathogens. Moreover, the transplant recipients may have been at greater risk for cancer for other reasons. For example, one oft-quoted study showed that patients who received heart transplants had rates of lung cancer that were 25 times those of the general population. This would seem to suggest that immunosuppression to pre-vent rejection of a transplanted heart increases the risk for cancer. However, individuals who received other types of transplants (e.g., kidneys), and who also were immu-nosuppressed, did not experience increased rates of lung cancer. Consequently, the increase in lung cancer in the heart transplant patients might simply reflect the fact that many of the patients in this study were cigarette smokers. So one must be careful in interpreting the results of stud-ies of cancer in immunosuppressed humans.

The important question to answer is this: **Does the immune system of a healthy human provide significant** protection against precancerous cells which would otherwise develop into cancers? To try to answer this question, let's examine the roles which various immune system cells might play in cancer surveillance – keeping in mind that their ability to provide meaningful surveillance may depend critically on the type of cancer.

CTLs and spontaneous tumors

The majority of human cancers are spontaneous tumors that are not of blood cell origin. It has been proposed that killer T cells might provide surveillance against these solid tumors. Let's try to evaluate this possibility.

The activation problem

Imagine that a heavy smoker finally accumulates enough mutations in the cells of his lungs to turn one of them into a cancer cell. Remember, it only takes one bad cell to make a cancer. And let's suppose that because of these mutations, this cell expresses proteins that could be recognized as foreign by CTLs. Now let me ask you a question: Where are this man's naive T cells while the tumor is growing in his lung? That's right. They are circulating through the blood, lymph, and secondary lymphoid organs. Do they leave this circulation pattern to enter the tissues of the lung? No, not until after they have been activated.

So right away, in terms of immune surveillance, we have a "traffic problem." To make self tolerance work, Mother Nature set up the traffic system so that naive T cells don't get out into the tissues where they might encounter self antigens that were not present in the thymus during tolerance induction. As a result, it's unlikely that virgin T cells ever would "see" tumor antigens expressed in the lung – because they just don't go there. **What we have here is a serious conflict between the need to preserve tolerance of self (and avoid autoimmune disease) and the need to provide surveillance against tumors that arise, as most tumors do, out in the tissues. And tolerance wins.**

Now, sometimes virgin T cells do disobey the traffic laws and wander out into the tissues. So you might imagine that this kind of adventure could give some T cells a chance to look at the tumor that's growing in this guy's lung, and be activated. But wait! What is required for T cell activation? First of all, killer T cells must recognize antigens which are produced within a cell and presented by class I MHC molecules on the surface of that cell. This means that the tumor cell itself must do the antigen presentation. So far, so good. However, CTLs also require co-stimulation from the cell that presents the antigen. Is this lung tumor cell going to provide that co-stimulation? I don't think so! This isn't an antigen presenting cell, after all. It's a plain old lung cell, and lung cells usually don't express co-stimulatory molecules like B7. Consequently, if a renegade, virgin CTL breaks the traffic laws, enters the lung, and recognizes a tumor antigen displayed by class I MHC molecules on the tumor cell, that CTL most likely will be anergized or killed – because the tumor cell will not provide the co-stimulation the CTL needs for survival.

Again we see a conflict between tolerance induction and tumor surveillance. **The two-key system of specific recognition plus co-stimulation was set up so that T cells which recognize self antigens out in the tissues, but which do not receive proper co-stimulation, will be anergized or killed to prevent autoimmunity. Unfortunately, this same two-key system makes it very difficult for CTLs to be activated by tumor cells that arise in the tissues. So the bottom line is that a CTL would have to perform "unnatural acts" to be activated by a tumor out in the tissues: It would have to break the traffic laws, and somehow avoid being anergized or killed. This could happen, of course, but it would be very inefficient compared to the activation of CTLs in response to, for example, a viral infection.

You might ask, "Why did Mother Nature put such a premium on avoiding autoimmune disease that she compromised the immune system's ability to defend against cancer?" What we need to remember is that the immune system did not evolve to protect people living in a modern society. It evolved to protect cavemen. Cancer was not a major worry for cavemen. They simply didn't live long enough to have a high probability of contracting this disease. So for them, a system that sacrificed a robust defense against cancer in favor of protection against autoimmune disease (which can be devastating to a young person) made perfect sense.

The mutation problem

Another possible scenario is that cancer cells from the primary tumor might metastasize to a lymph node, where T cells could be activated. However, by the time this happens, the original tumor probably will have become quite large. Even a tumor that weighs only about half an ounce will contain more than 10 billion cancer cells – more cells than there are people on our planet! This poses a major problem for immune surveillance, because cancer cells usually mutate like crazy, and with so many cells mutating, it is likely that some of these mutations will prevent recognition or presentation of tumor antigens. For example, the gene encoding the tumor antigen itself might mutate so that the tumor antigen no longer can be recognized by activated CTLs, or no longer will fit properly into the groove of an MHC molecule for presentation. In addition, tumor cells can mutate so that they stop producing the particular MHC molecules that CTLs are restricted to recognize. This happens quite frequently: About 15% of the tumors that have been examined have lost expression of at least one of their MHC molecules. Also, genes that encode the TAP transporters can mutate in a tumor cell, with the result that tumor antigens will not be efficiently transported for loading onto class I MHC molecules. Indeed, a **tumor cell's high mutation rate is its greatest advantage over the immune system, and usually keeps these cells one step ahead of surveillance by CTLs.**

Cancer cells fight back

We have discussed how difficult it is for cells, when they first become cancerous, to activate the adaptive immune system. Nevertheless, when some solid tumors are removed from patients late in the disease, immunologists have discovered that these cancers have been infiltrated by tumor-specific CTLs. This begs the question: Why don't these CTLs destroy the tumors in these patients?

We have already discussed part of the answer to this question. Although these killer T cells may recognize and kill some of the cancer cells, other cells in the growing tumor likely will have mutated so that they cannot be recognized by the killer T cells which have been activated. In addition, tumor-specific CTLs face yet another problem: Cancer cells fight back. Once a solid tumor has been established, the cancer cells can modify the environment in the neighborhood of the tumor to make it more difficult for tumor-specific CTLs to operate.

In Lecture 8, I mentioned two inhibitory receptors, CTLA-4 and PD-1, which are found on the surface of activated T cells. The natural function of these **checkpoint proteins** is to restrain CTLs so that the immune response does not become overexuberant. However, many types of cancer cells express the ligands for these immunosuppressive proteins, and the ligation of CTLA-4 and/or PD-1 on tumor-specific killer T cells can impair their function. The result is that the growing tumor is able to "shield" itself from killing by tumor-specific CTLs. Tumor immunologists have now treated patients with antibodies that block the interaction between these two inhibitory receptors and their ligands. Early results from these clinical trials suggest that such **immune checkpoint inhibitors** can be useful in helping CTLs deal with established tumors.

Many tumors express high levels of the enzyme **indoleamine 2,3-dioxygenase (IDO)**. This enzyme catalyzes the metabolism of the essential amino acid tryptophan, resulting in the rapid consumption of tryptophan from the tumor environment. And when killer T cells are starved for tryptophan, they stop proliferating and become anergic. Also, tumor cells can increase the production of Treg cells in their neighborhood. Exactly how this is accomplished is not well understood, but the result is that Tregs secrete TGF-β and IL-10, creating an immunosuppressive environment in which CTLs function poorly.

My conclusion is that **killer T cells provide limited protection against solid tumors when these cells first become cancerous – because CTLs are inefficiently activated early in the course of the disease. Later, when the tumor becomes large, killer T cells may be activated. However, at this late stage, CTLs are relatively ineffective at eradicating the tumor: The high mutation rate of the cells in the tumor allows them to escape immunosurveillance, and the tumor creates an immunosuppresive environment which blunts the effectiveness of tumor-specific killer T cells. Consequently, even when it occurs, CTL surveillance against solid tumors usually is a case of "too little, too late."**

CTLs and cancerous blood cells

Okay, so CTLs probably don't provide serious surveillance against non-blood cell, spontaneous tumors, especially when they first arise. That's a real bummer, because these make up the majority of human tumors. But what about blood cell cancers like leukemia and lymphoma? Maybe CTLs are useful against them. After all, immunosuppressed humans do have higher frequencies of leukemia and lymphoma than do humans with healthy immune systems. This suggests that there might be something fundamentally different about the way the immune system views tumors in tissues and organs versus the way it sees blood cells that have become cancerous. Let's take a look at what these differences might be.

One of the problems that CTLs have in providing surveillance against tumors that arise in tissues is that these tumors simply are not on the normal traffic pattern of virgin T cells – and it's hard to imagine how a CTL could be activated by a cancer it doesn't see. In contrast, most blood cell cancers are found in the blood, lymph, and secondary lymphoid organs, and this is ideal for viewing by CTLs, which pass through these areas all the time. Thus, in the case of blood cell cancers, the traffic patterns of cancer cells and virgin T cells actually intersect. Moreover, in contrast to tumors in tissues, which usually are unable to supply the co-stimulation required for activation of virgin T cells, some cancerous blood cells actually express high levels of B7, and therefore can provide the necessary co-stimulation. These properties of blood cell cancers suggest that CTLs may provide surveillance against some of them. Unfortunately, this surveillance must be incomplete, because people with otherwise healthy immune systems still get leukemias and lymphomas.

CTLs and virus-associated tumors

Certain viral infections can predispose a person to particular types of cancer. Because Mother Nature designed killer T cells to defend against viral infections, it is easy to imagine that CTLs might provide surveillance against virus-associated tumors. Unfortunately, this surveillance is probably quite limited. Here's why.

Most viruses cause "acute" infections in which all the virus-infected cells are rather quickly destroyed by the immune system. And because a dead cell isn't going to make a tumor, **viruses which only cause acute infections do not play a role in cancer.** This explains why most viral infections are <u>not</u> associated with human cancer.

There are viruses, however, which can evade the immune system and cause long-term (sometimes lifelong) infections. Indeed, **all viruses which have been shown to play a role in causing cancer are able to establish long-lasting infections during which they "hide" from the immune system.** However, CTLs cannot destroy virus-infected cells while they are hiding, and because these hidden cells are the very ones which eventually become cancerous, it can be argued that CTLs do not provide effective surveillance against virus-associated cancer.

Of course, you might propose that without killer T cells, more cells would be infected during a virus attack, thereby increasing the number of cells in which the virus might be able to establish a long-term, hidden infection. And this probably is true. In fact, this may help explain why humans with deficient immune systems have higher than normal rates of virus-associated tumors. However, the bottom line is that **CTLs cannot provide significant surveillance against virus-infected cells once they have become cancerous, because these cancers only result from long-term viral infections – infections which CTLs cannot detect or cannot deal with effectively.**

IMMUNE SURVEILLANCE BY MACROPHAGES AND NK CELLS

Macrophages and natural killer cells may provide surveillance against some cancers. Hyperactivated macrophages secrete TNF, and express it on their surface. Either form of TNF can kill certain types of tumor cells in the test tube. This brings up an important point: **What happens in the test tube is not always the same as what happens in an animal.** For example, there are mouse sarcoma cells that are very resistant to killing by TNF in the test tube. In contrast, when live mice that have these same sarcomas are treated with TNF, their tumors are rapidly destroyed. Studies of this phenomenon showed that the reason TNF is able to kill the tumor when it is in the animal is that this cytokine actually attacks the blood vessels that feed the tumor, cutting off the blood supply and causing the tumor cells to starve to death. This type of death is called necrosis, and it was this observation that led scientists to name this cytokine "tumor necrosis factor."

In humans, there are examples of cancer therapies in which activated macrophages are likely to play a major role in tumor rejection. One such therapy involves injecting the tumor with **bacille Calmette–Guérin (BCG)**, a cousin of the bacterium that causes tuberculosis. BCG hyperactivates macrophages, and when it is injected directly into a tumor (e.g., a melanoma), the tumor fills up with highly activated macrophages that can destroy the cancer. In fact, one way of treating bladder cancer is to inject it with BCG – a treatment which is quite effective in eliminating superficial tumors, probably through the action of hyperactivated macrophages.

But how do macrophages tell the difference between normal cells and cancer cells? The answer to this question is not known for certain, but evidence suggests that macrophages recognize tumor cells that have unusual cell surface molecules. One of the duties of macrophages in the spleen is to test red blood cells to see if they have been damaged or are old. Macrophages use their sense of "feel" to determine which red cells are past their prime. And when they find an old one, they eat it. What macrophages feel for is a fat molecule called phosphatidylserine. This particular fat is usually found on the inside of young red blood cells, but flips to the outside when the cells get old. Like old red blood cells, tumor cells also tend to have unusual surface molecules, and in fact, some express phosphatidylserine on their surface. It is believed that **the abnormal expression of surface molecules on** tumor cells may allow activated macrophages to differentiate between cancer cells and normal cells.

Natural killer cells target cells that express low levels of class I MHC molecules, and which display unusual surface molecules (e.g., proteins which indicate that the target cells are "stressed"). In the test tube, natural killer cells can destroy some tumor cells. In addition, there is evidence that NK cells can kill cancer cells in the body. Certainly, there would be a number of advantages to having macrophages and NK cells provide surveillance against wannabe cancer cells. First, unlike CTLs, which take a week or more to get cranked up, macrophages and NK cells are quick-acting. This is an important consideration, because the longer abnormal cells have to proliferate, the greater is the likelihood they will mutate to take on the characteristics of metastatic cancer cells. In addition, once a tumor becomes large, it is much more difficult for the immune system to deal with. So you would like the weapons that protect against cancer cells to be ready to go just as soon as the cells start to get a little weird.

You would also like anti-tumor weapons to be focused on diverse targets, because a single target (e.g., the MHC–peptide combination seen by a killer T cell) can be mutated, rendering the target unrecognizable. Both NK cells and macrophages recognize diverse target structures, so the chances of them being fooled by a single mutation is small. In addition, macrophages are located out in the tissues where most tumors arise, so they can intercept cancer cells at an early stage. And with immune surveillance, as with real estate, location is everything.

There are problems, however, with macrophages and NK cells providing surveillance against cancer. Macrophages need to be hyperactivated before they can kill cancer cells. That's what the BCG treatments do: They hyperactivate macrophages by causing inflammation. So if a wannabe cancer cell arises at a site of inflammation where macrophages are already hyperactivated, that's great. But if there's no inflammatory reaction going on, macrophages will probably remain in a resting state and simply ignore the cancer cells. Unlike macrophages, which are found in large numbers in our tissues, most NK cells are found in the blood. Like neutrophils, NK cells are "on call." And the cells which do the calling are activated macrophages and dendritic cells that are responding to an invasion. So again, unless there is an inflammatory reaction going on in the tissues, most NK cells will just continue to circulate in the blood.

As a tumor grows, it eventually becomes so large that the neighboring blood vessels cannot provide the nutri-

ents and oxygen required for continued growth, and some of the cancer cells begin to die. Cancer cells also die when they accumulate mutations that are lethal. Consequently, at a later stage in the growth of a tumor, dying cancer cells may provide the signals required to activate macrophages – which can then recruit natural killer cells from the blood. So at this point, macrophages and NK cells may play a role in destroying at least some of the tumor cells. In addition, because NK cells do not need to be activated to kill, natural killer cells that are circulating in the blood may be able to destroy either blood cell cancers or cancer cells that are metastasizing through the blood from a primary tumor.

VACCINATION TO PREVENT VIRUS-ASSOCIATED CANCER

One approach which has been successful in using the immune system to prevent cancer is vaccination against tumor viruses. A chronic infection with hepatitis B virus increases one's risk of getting liver cancer about 200-fold, and roughly 20% of long-term hepatitis B carriers eventually develop this disease. Moreover, hepatitis B virus ranks as one of the most infectious of all viruses: Transfer of a fraction of a drop of blood is sufficient to spread the virus from one human to another. Fortunately, vaccines that protect against infection by hepatitis B virus have been available in the United States since 1982, and the current vaccine is administered not only to healthcare professionals who routinely come into contact with blood and blood products, but also to children. This subunit vaccine gives the immune system a "preview" of a real hepatitis B infection, allowing ample time for memory B cells and the antibodies they produce to be mobilized. If infection does occur, the prepared immune system can quickly eradicate the virus, effectively preventing hepatitis B-associated liver cancer.

Infection with certain "oncogenic" types of human papillomavirus (HPV) can increase the risk of cervical cancer. These viruses are spread by sexual contact, and there are now so many women infected with this virus that cervical carcinoma has become the second most common cancer in women worldwide, resulting in about 250 000 deaths per year.

Although there are about a dozen slightly different types of HPV that are associated with cervical cancer, two types, HPV-16 and HPV-18, are implicated in about 70% of all cervical cancer cases. Two pharmaceutical companies, Merck and GSK, have pioneered vaccines that are effective in preventing infection by both types of HPV. These are subunit vaccines made from viral coat proteins. In addition, the Merck vaccine includes coat proteins from two other HPV types, HPV-6 and HPV-11, which are not associated with cervical cancer, but which do cause genital warts in both men and women. Their thinking in including these two "extras" is that preventing genital warts might encourage boys and men to be vaccinated, since they might otherwise be reluctant to be vaccinated to prevent a disease (cervical cancer) they cannot get.

Although the Merck and GSK vaccines will be very helpful in decreasing the number of deaths from cervical cancer, a vaccine that would protect against all five HPV types most commonly associated with cervical carcinoma could prevent hundreds of thousands of deaths from cancer each year – providing that most sexually active young women could be vaccinated. Unfortunately, many of the cases of cervical cancer occur in underdeveloped parts of the world, where immunization via injection is problematic.

REVIEW

Although it is certain that human cells have built-in safeguards to protect them from becoming cancerous, it is not nearly so clear what role the immune system plays in protecting us against this terrible disease. The immune system probably is able to defend against some virus-associated and blood cell cancers. Also, natural killer cells and macrophages can recognize and kill some tumor cells – those which have unusual molecules on their surface. And NK cells may reduce the frequency of metastases or help slow the metastatic process once a primary tumor has formed. Consequently, macrophages and NK cells may be useful against certain types of cancer. However, it is unlikely that killer T cells provide significant surveillance against most solid tumors in humans. There are several reasons for this.

First there is the activation problem. Many safeguards are in place to protect humans against autoimmunity, and these safeguards make it very difficult for cancer-specific CTLs to be activated – especially during the early stages of tumor development. Virgin T cells are activated in the secondary lymphoid organs. Consequently, the normal traffic pattern of naive T cells keeps them from coming in contact with cancer cells in the tissues. In addition, most cancer cells cannot supply the co-stimulation required to activate killer T cells, so even a "chance encounter" between a naive T cell and a tumor cell out in the tissues isn't likely to result in activation.

Another obstacle to cancer surveillance by killer T cells is that, because of their high mutation rate, cancer cells represent a "moving target." Even if a CTL can be activated so that it can attack some cells in a tumor, it is very likely that there will be other cancer cells within that tumor which have mutated so that they are invisible to that killer T cell. In addition, once a tumor becomes large, the rapidly mutating tumor cells create an immunosuppressive environment. And this can blunt the immune response and make CTLs ineffective.

Vaccination against infection by cancer-associated viruses is the current star in the effort to enlist the immune system in the battle against cancer. However, many other approaches are in various stages of testing. We all can hope that these experiments will be successful – because, as it stands now, about one out of every three of us will get cancer during our lifetime.

THOUGHT QUESTIONS

1. There is a conflict between immune surveillance against cancer and the preservation of tolerance of self antigens. Explain.

2. Discuss why the adaptive immune system may provide some surveillance against blood cell cancers, but not against spontaneous, non-blood cell cancers.

3. Why can macrophages and NK cells only be expected to destroy cancer cells under special circumstances?

4. Vaccines against tumor viruses can help prevent virus-associated cancer. What obstacles to you foresee which might make it difficult for immunologists to make vaccines that would prevent other forms of cancer?

Glossary

Adjuvant: A vaccine component included to increase its potency.

Allergen: An antigen that causes allergies.

Anergize: To render non-functional.

Anergy: A state of non-functionality.

Antibody-dependent cellular cytotoxicity: Antibodies form a "bridge" between the target and the cytotoxic cell. Antibody-directed killing by cells of the innate system.

Antigen: A rather loosely used term for the target (e.g., a viral protein) of an antibody or a T cell. To be more precise, an antibody binds to a <u>region</u> of an antigen called the epitope, and the T cell receptor binds to a peptide that is a <u>fragment</u> of an antigen.

Antigen presenting cells: Cells that can present antigen efficiently to T cells via MHC molecules, and which can supply the co-stimulatory molecules required to activate T cells.

Apoptosis: The process during which a cell commits suicide in response to problems within the cell or to signals from outside the cell.

Atopic individual: Someone who has allergies.

Autophagy: A process by which starved cells recycle their components.

β2-microglobulin: The non-polymorphic chain of the class I MHC molecule.

Central tolerance induction: The process by which T cells with receptors that recognize abundant self antigens in the thymus are anergized or deleted.

Checkpoint proteins: Proteins such as CTLA-4 and PD-1 which help turn off the immune system once an invasion has been repulsed.

Chemokine: A special cytokine used to direct cells to their proper positions.

Clonal selection principle: When receptors on B or T cells recognize their cognate antigen, these cells are triggered (selected) to proliferate. As a result, a clone of B or T cells with identical antigen specificities is produced.

Cognate antigen: The antigen (e.g., a bacterial protein) which a B or T cell's receptors recognize and bind to.

Colon: A synonym for large intestine.

Commensal bacteria: Bacteria that have a beneficial, symbiotic relationship with their host.

Co-receptor: The CD4 or CD8 molecules on T cells, or the complement receptor on B cells.

Cortical thymic epithelial cells: Cells in the cortex of the thymus which are the "examiners" during positive selection (MHC restriction) of T cells.

Co-stimulation: The second "key" that B and T cells need for activation.

Crosslink: Cluster together (e.g., an antigen may crosslink a B cell's receptors).

Cross reacts: Recognizes several different epitopes. For example, a B cell's receptors may bind to (cross react with) several different epitopes.

Cytokine profile: The mixture of different cytokines that a cell secretes.

Cytokines: Hormone-like messenger molecules that cells use to communicate.

Cytotoxic lymphocyte: A synonym for killer T cell.

Delayed-type hypersensitivity: An inflammatory reaction in which Th cells recognize a specific invader, and secrete cytokines that activate and recruit innate system cells to do the killing.

Dendritic cell: A starfish-shaped cell which, when activated by battle signals, travels from the tissues to the secondary lymphoid organs to activate naive T cells.

Elite controller: A rare, untreated, AIDS patient whose immune system is able to control his or her viral load so that it remains low for an extended period.

Endogenous protein: A protein that is produced within the cell in question – the opposite of an exogenous protein.

Endoplasmic reticulum: A large sack-like structure inside a cell from which most proteins destined for transport to the cell surface begin their journey.

Endothelial cells: Cells shaped like shingles which line the inside of our blood vessels.

Epithelial cells: Cells that form part of the barrier that separates your body from the outside world.

Epitope: The region of an antigen that is recognized by a B or T cell's receptors.

Exogenous protein: A protein that is found outside the cell in question – the opposite of an endogenous protein.

f-met peptide: A peptide which includes a special initiator amino acid that is characteristic of proteins made by bacteria.

Follicular dendritic cell: A starfish-shaped cell which retains opsonized antigens in germinal centers, and displays these antigens to help activate B cells.

Follicular helper T cell: A helper T cell which has been "licensed" to provide help to B cells in germinal centers.

Germinal center: An area in a secondary lymphoid organ in which B cells proliferate, undergo somatic hypermutation, and switch classes.

Granzyme B: An enzyme which CTLs and NK cells use to destroy their targets.

High endothelial venule: A region in a blood vessel where there are high endothelial cells which allow lymphocytes to exit the blood.

Inducible regulatory T cells: CD4$^+$ T cells which produce cytokines that suppress the immune response to invaders.

Inflammatory response: A rather general term that describes the battle that macrophages, neutrophils, and other immune system cells wage against an invader.

Interferon alpha and beta: Warning cytokines secreted by virus-infected cells.

Interferon gamma: A battle cytokine secreted mainly by Th1 helper T cells and NK cells.

Interleukin: A protein (cytokine) that is used for communication between leukocytes.

Intestinal microbiota: All the microbes in the intestines.

Invariant chain: A small protein which occupies the binding groove of a class II MHC molecule until it is replaced by an exogenous peptide.

Isotype: A synonym for class. The isotype of an antibody (e.g., IgA or IgG) is determined by the constant region of its heavy chain.

Lamina propria: The tissues that surround the small and large intestine.

Leukocytes: A generic term that includes all of the different kinds of white blood cells.

Ligand: A molecule that binds to a receptor (e.g., the Fas ligand binds to the Fas receptor protein on the surface of a cell).

Ligate: Bind to. When a receptor has bound its ligand, the receptor is said to be ligated.

Lipopolysaccharide: A component of the outer membrane of many bacteria. It serves as a "danger signal" for the innate immune system.

Lymph: The liquid that "leaks" out of blood vessels into the tissues.

Lymphocyte: The generic term for a B cell or a T cell.

Lymphoid follicle: The region of a secondary lymphoid organ that contains follicular dendritic cells embedded in a sea of B cells.

M cell: A cell that crowns a Peyer's patch, and which specializes in sampling antigen from the intestine.

Medullary thymic epithelial cell: A cell found in the medulla of the thymus which expresses tissue-specific self antigens, and which takes part in the examination of T cells for tolerance of self antigens (negative selection).

MHC proteins: Proteins encoded by the major histocompatibility complex (a chromosomal region that includes a "complex" of genes involved in antigen presentation).

MHC restriction: Survival in the thymus is restricted to T cells whose receptors recognize MHC–self antigen complexes (a synonym for positive selection).

Microbe: A generic term which includes bacteria, viruses, fungi, and parasites.

Mitogen: A molecule that can cause the polyclonal activation of B cells.

Monocytes: White blood cells that are the precursors of macrophages or dendritic cells.

Mucosa: The tissues and associated mucus that protect exposed surfaces such as the gastrointestinal and respiratory tracts.

Mucosal-associated lymphoid tissues: Secondary lymphoid organs that are associated with mucosa (e.g., Peyer's patches and tonsils).

Naive lymphocytes: B or T cells which have never been activated.

Natural regulatory T cells: CD4$^+$ T cells that are selected in the thymus and which negatively regulate the immune response by interfering with the activation of self-reactive T cells in the secondary lymphoid organs.

Necrosis: Cell death, typically caused by burns or other trauma. This type of cell death (as opposed to apoptotic cell death) usually results in the contents of the cell being dumped into the tissues.

Negative selection: Synonym for central tolerance induction. The selection of T cells whose receptors do not recognize MHC–self peptide complexes in the thymus.

Neutralizing antibody: An antibody which can bind to a pathogen, and prevent it from infecting or reproducing in the cells it would like to infect.

Opsonize: To "decorate" with fragments of complement proteins or with antibodies.

Pathogen: A disease-causing agent (e.g., a bacterium or a virus).

Peptide: A small fragment of a protein, usually only tens of amino acids in length.

Perforin: A molecule used by CTLs and NK cells to help destroy their targets.

Peripheral tolerance induction: The mechanisms that induce self tolerance outside of the thymus.

Phagocytes: Cells such as macrophages and neutrophils that engulf (phagocytose) invaders.

Plasma B cells: B cells which produce a large burst of antibodies in response to an attack, and then die.

Polyclonal activation: Activation of many B cells with different specificities.

Positive selection: A synonym for MHC restriction.

Primary lymphoid organs: The thymus and the bone marrow.

Proliferate: Increase in number. A cell proliferates by dividing into two daughter cells, which then can divide again to give four cells, and so on. Cellular reproduction.

Proteasome: A multi-protein complex in the cell that chops up proteins into small pieces.

Receptor editing: The process by which B cells in the bone marrow can "draw again from the deck" to try to make a BCR that is not self-reactive.

Secondary lymphoid organs: Organs such as lymph nodes, Peyer's patches, and the spleen in which activation of naive B and T cells takes place.

Secrete: Export out of the cell (e.g., cytokines are secreted by the T cells that produce them, and antibodies are secreted by B cells).

Thymic dendritic cell: A cell found in the medulla of the thymus which tests T cells for tolerance of self antigens (negative selection).

Tolerance: Not viewing self as an attacker.

Tolerize: To make B cells and T cells tolerant of our self antigens.

Toll-like receptors: Receptor molecules found on the surface of cells or inside cells. These receptors have evolved to recognize the signatures of common invaders, and to generate signals which alert the immune system to danger.

Tumor necrosis factor: A battle cytokine secreted mainly by macrophages and helper T cells.

Virgin lymphocyte: A B or T cell which has never been activated. A synonym for naive lymphocyte.

List of Acronyms and Abbreviations

ADCC: Antibody-dependent cellular cytotoxicity

APC: Antigen presenting cell

BCR: B cell receptor

cTEC: Cortical thymic epithelial cell

CTL: Cytotoxic lymphocyte

DAF: Decay accelerating factor

DAMP: Damage-associated molecular pattern

DC: Dendritic cell

DTH: Delayed-type hypersensitivity

ER: Endoplasmic reticulum

Fab: Antigen-binding fragment of an antibody molecule

FasL: Fas ligand

Fc: Constant fragment of an antibody molecule

FDC: Follicular dendritic cell

Hc: Heavy chain protein of an antibody molecule

HEV: High endothelial venule

IFN: Interferon, as in IFN-α

IgG: Immunoglobulin G

IL: Interleukin, as in IL-1

iTreg: Inducible regulatory T cell

Lc: Light chain protein of an antibody molecule

LPS: Lipopolysaccharide

MAC: Membrane attack complex

MALT: Mucosal-associated lymphoid tissue

MBL: Mannose-binding lectin

MHC: Major histocompatibility complex

mTEC: Medullary thymic epithelial cell

NK: Natural killer, as in NK cell

nTreg: Natural regulatory T cell

PALS: Periarteriolar lymphocyte sheath

PAMP: Pathogen-associated molecular pattern

PD-1: Programmed death 1

PD-1L: The ligand for PD-1

pDC: Plasmacytoid dendritic cell

PRR: Pattern-recognition receptor

SCIDS: Severe combined immunodeficiency syndrome

TCR: T cell receptor

TDC: Thymic dendritic cell

Tfh cell: Follicular helper T cell

Th cell: Helper T cell

TLR: Toll-like receptor

TNF: Tumor necrosis factor

How the Immune System Works, Fifth Edition. Lauren Sompayrac. © 2016 John Wiley & Sons, Ltd. Published 2016 by John Wiley & Sons, Ltd.

Index